CANCER
TIME
BOMB

HOW THE BRCA GENE
STOLE MY TITS AND EGGS

JOELLE B. BURNETTE

Cancer Time Bomb:
How the BRCA Genetic Mutation Stole My Tits and Eggs

By Joelle Burnette

Copyright © 2012 Joelle Burnette

First Edition.

ISBN 978-1475152210

~~~~~~~~~~~~~~~~

This book is dedicated to

my mom who displays boundless support, strength,

love and friendship,

and to

Michelle, my incredibly brave sister.

~~~~~~~~~~~~~~~

ACKNOWLEDGMENTS

When times get difficult, my mom always says, "God will provide."
Mom knows I'm more of a believer in fate, rather than faith,
so here are some of the people who have been blessings in my life
and at just the right time during my BRCA journey:

Mark, my patient, loving husband who keeps me laughing.
My mench of a son and
my lovely daughter who brings a smile to my face.

My supportive family and friends:
Dad, Donna & Bill, Syl & Bert,
Brita & Chuck, "Lilly," Min, Stephie, Janice K.
Melody O., Kim W., Karen W., Cheryl J., Sheila A.,
Susan A., Jan F., Connie H.,
Shari K., Judy D., Laura A., Nancy S., Rikki F., Rabbi G.

Special thanks to the many people at
UCSF Medical Center (Mount Zion Hospital)
who offered kindness, patience and guidance.

Many thanks.
J

CHAPTER 1:
LIGHTNING STRIKES TWICE

Waiting for the school day to end, I sat outside my daughter's classroom expecting the bell to ring at any moment. The door would swing open, and her first-grade teacher would stand in the entryway handing out colorful notes shaped like stars to students who had a good day in class. I hoped Sophie was among those children although it wasn't always the case.

I had found a shady spot and enjoyed the warm Sonoma County day. I was chatting with another mother when my cell phone rang and displayed "Mom" on the screen.

"Hi, mom." I answered my phone expecting her usual questions about what I was up to; what had I taught in art at my children's school that day, and how her grandbabies were doing? Maybe she'd offer news about my dad's health that has been deteriorating exponentially after years of battling diabetes.

"Joey," she said through tears.

"Mom, what's wrong?" Immediately, I assumed dad was in the hospital again, or worse.

At first, she couldn't speak. Finally, she said, "It's your sister. She...." I couldn't hear the end of her sentence because the school bell suddenly shrieked across the campus announcing the end of the school day.

"What? Wait, mom, I can't hear you. The bell...." I spoke loudly into the phone. The school bell seemed to ring forever. She was talking, but I couldn't make out what she was saying through all the commotion as the formerly peaceful corridor between the rows of classrooms flooded with children and parents.

"What did you say?" I asked while firmly pressing the mobile

1

phone against my right ear. I held my free hand over my left ear trying to block out the cacophony.

"The cancer is back," she cried.

"What?" I responded in shock. "But it's been...," *think, think,* "It's been more than 10 years." I couldn't believe this horrible news. My mind was racing, flashing back to my sister's frail body all those years ago when our family feared she was going to die.

The first time Michelle had breast cancer in 1994, it took forever for her private health insurance to approve any tests and treatments.

At the time, she was only 32. Her health insurance (an HMO) was convinced the lump in her breast was nothing more than fatty tissue; perhaps a cyst. But certainly not breast cancer. She was too young to be struck by the disease.

Yes, the anonymous desk jockey from her insurance company insisted this was the case simply by talking with Michelle over the phone when my sister tried to secure appropriate medical attention and treatment. It seemed they'd rather she drop dead than cover the expense of a mammogram and related tests.

Ladies, you know when you go to the gynecologist's office, and sitting on the table is that fake boob containing various types of tumors? You're supposed to feel it, press into the lumps. By doing so, you learn what to detect when carrying out self-exams. My sister had the marble-hard lump. The one you try to squeeze between your fingers as if you're going to get a prize if it pops out of the gelatinous mass.

I remember that day at my parent's house when my sister asked if I would feel an unexpected bulge in her breast. She wanted my opinion of whether or not she should be concerned. Upon barely pressing my fingers into her skin, I swiftly recoiled my hand as though I was instinctively protecting myself from getting burned.

"Yes, you need to make an appointment right away," I told her. "Michelle, that's precisely what they tell you to look for when you're feeling your boobs."

Several months would pass before she received approval for medical attention, and only after having hired an attorney who specialized in this type of "HMO wants to fuck you out of treatment that will save your life" case and threatening lawsuits. By that time, the original tumor in her breast had doubled in size and the cancer metastasized into 14 lymph nodes in her armpit.

Ultimately, she was diagnosed with an aggressive, Stage 3 breast cancer.

The impassive assumption made by her HMO was wrong. By the time she got an appointment to see an oncologist, she was told she'd be lucky to have six months to live. She should put her life in order, make any necessary arrangements. Perhaps, travel.

Michelle's spirit was beaten down by horrible months filled with chemotherapy treatments accompanied by an onslaught of puking. All the while, our parents refused to allow cancer to kill their daughter, or her spirit; both were tormented by cancer's dark grip. Ultimately, their determination to keep Michelle alive ensured her survival.

Dark rings bordered my sister's eyes while her body was repeatedly butchered by surgeries and other forms of torture including a bone marrow transplant: an agonizing, long process that left her body weak and forever after impacted by unforgiving side effects.

Fuck you, doctor doom. Michelle beat the odds and became a breast cancer survivor. Not someone who becomes a warm and fuzzy "I'm going to tell my story at every cancer walk I can find" survivor; simply a woman who survived a process through which no person should have to suffer. (I have nothing against women who tell their story. These stories are necessary to get men off their asses to realize women's healthcare issues are important and require progressive action. Still, I don't think my sister's personality fits the breast cancer poster package.)

Michelle survived so she could continue trying to find her place in the world. She could figure out what to do with a future she thought was being ripped away too early in her already challenging life.

Oh, and thanks to the American healthcare system and all its presumptuous delays, one of the HMO's parting gifts was the enormous bill she (actually, mostly our parents) had to pay in return for this new gift of life.

Along her cancer journey, she and my parents met ample number of people who weren't as lucky because they had no money for the expensive medicines required to survive. Those were the people the system left for dead.

Still, after every medical treatment was completed (except radiation; she turned that down) and she survived suffering through each step, the last note of dreadful news came at the end. The doctors' message was clear. If Michelle's cancer ever returned, there was nothing more they could do for her.

For years, that message weighed heavily on all of us; heaviest on my parents who already felt guilty about Michelle's difficult childhood.

Learning disabilities and her demanding temperament had plagued my sister's youth before she became a generally lonely adult. She's not the easiest person to get along with. She has a short shelf life when visiting with family who know her well, let alone spending time with others.

Add cancer to that recipe and you wonder why some people get handed one piece of shitty news after another while others rarely deal with any worries.

Once the cancer was sliced away and killed by chemicals, Michelle's life appeared to be changing for the better. Regardless, my parents quietly planned for the worst and told Michelle to follow her desires: travel abroad, try to get one of her many screenplays produced while she lived in Los Angeles, take some classes, have some fun.

Always, those bucket list items were accompanied by the whispered caveat, "do these things while you still can, before cancer tries to kill you again."

"Your sister's cancer can come back at any time," my mom reinforced every time Michelle found something new she wanted to try. "She's not going to live that long. Dad and I just want her to have something good in her life while she can."

Then, the day arrived when the doctor's death sentence—one that had been handed down more than a decade earlier—appeared imminent.

"But mom, they said if she ever got cancer again…," I could produce no more words. My head pulsed with pain. I felt I would fall over if I tried to stand.

"I know, Joey. I just wanted to tell you. I think you should start spending more time with your sister. Come down this weekend. Look, I have to go," she said through more tears; her voice producing a higher pitch as emotions took control of her words. We hung up.

Sophie exited her classroom and approached me with her usual smile. Thankfully, this wasn't a day the teacher needed to talk to me about her behavior in class.

My older son hadn't yet walked over from his fifth-grade classroom located down the next parallel corridor. Sophie and I walked to his class where Jesse was still in the room gathering his books and papers. I did what I could to hold in my emotions. *Hold it together, at least until we get home.*

A friend—another mom whose son was in Jesse's class—was inside chatting with the teacher. Our boys had known each other since first grade, and our daughters were best friends.

I was trying to rush Jesse along, but Clare finished speaking with the teacher. She looked at me, and when her expression changed, I realized, I must not be concealing my emotions well. She said with concern, "Are you okay?"

That's all it took. I broke down crying. I felt my face flush red and I couldn't get any words out. I could only wave my hands about as though that motion would help me to speak.

"I'm sorry," I could only manage. I began shaking uncontrollably. I tried hiding my face that contorted as I cried. I was glad most everyone had already left the school by then.

"What's wrong?" Clare and the teacher asked soothingly. They waited to hear what had left me exceedingly upset. Clare gently rubbed my back in a circular motion as though she were comforting a child.

"It's my sister," I finally said. "The cancer is back," I could only whisper.

Another parent entered the room. The teacher left our conversation to provide some privacy while drawing that mother away and over to the other side of the room. Clare remained by my side.

"Oh, no. It's *that* sister?" She recalled what I had told her about Michelle's health. Ironically, she and I had been speaking about my sister's cancer only a week prior while we were on a field trip with our kids.

"When she had cancer last time, the doctors said they wouldn't be able to do anything for her if she got it again because of all the chemo and the bone marrow transplant," I reminded her of my fears.

I can't lose another sister, became my mind's mantra. *I'll be all alone.* My eldest sister, Renee, had just turned 19 years old when she rode along as a passenger in a Volkswagen Bug belonging to one of her best friends; Renee was killed instantly in a car accident. I was

12 at the time.

The driver survived with a broken bone, but I've heard her life was essentially destroyed after that. I'm told she never made it through to the other side of the tragedy and for that, I pity her. Wasting a life is not what Renee would have wanted.

Clare wrapped her arms around me to give me a hug. "Well, then, there's nothing you can do." I couldn't believe she was giving up on my remaining sister's life so quickly.

Her cold response angered me, but I concealed my reaction by looking down. *What a shitty thing to say.* This isn't a pet you can take to the vet and put to sleep. This is a sister, a daughter. Her body was going to be poked and sliced and mutilated again, just to be told, there was nothing more they could do for her.

I listened to Clare's words that were meant to be supportive. Frustration settled into my brain as my heart ached because people just don't get it. They don't realize how horrible it is to lose someone so close and then be forced to face the news you may lose another loved one to a painful, useless death.

It appeared my life was about to be turned upside down again by another sister's death. I never fully recovered from Renee's death; and now, my only remaining sibling could be stolen from our family. Regardless of our complicated, difficult relationship, Michelle is still my sister. I *couldn't* lose her.

My friend offered kind words after her initial message to submit to death's bidding, but my head hurt too much and my stomach was too upset to remember anything else she said. I had to get home and talk with my family.

CHAPTER 2:
TAKE THE FUCKING TEST

We drove south to my parent's home in Marin County to visit with my sister who, it was decided, would not return to her home in Los Angeles. Rather, she would be staying with my parents the next several months while she went through chemotherapy, surgeries, and whatever else she needed to fight the new cancer.

Little more than a week before, Michelle had returned to Northern California to spend the holidays with our family. She was taking a shower at my parent's home when she felt a lump in her deceptively healthy breast.

She made an appointment through the Veterans Affairs (VA) hospital in San Francisco to see a nurse practitioner who immediately sent her less than four miles away to the Carol Franc Buck Breast Care Center at University of California, San Francisco Medical Center at Mount Zion on Divisadero Street. (For future reference, I refer to this location as the cancer center, the Breast Care Center, Mount Zion, or simply UCSF). Because of her medical history, Michelle was seen immediately at Mount Zion.

In one day, a Monday, she had a mammogram, more tests, a biopsy and the diagnosis of Stage 1 breast cancer. By Friday that same week, she received the first round of chemotherapy after having a surgery to implant a portal in her chest.

We were amazed by the advances that had been made during the decade that had passed. For instance, we waited for the vomiting to begin, but mostly, it didn't (other than some minimal barfing).

The first time around, Michelle (or my mom) had to carry a bucket most places. This time, she rarely felt nauseated by the medicine.

Moreover, while my parents had to use every possible motivation to peel Michelle's weak body off the couch more than a decade prior, now her hyperactive energy rarely waned.

Still, one thing that did stay the same was the general bickering between my sister and parents (and with me).

"I don't know why you didn't just take off the other breast the first time. I would have taken off the other breast," my mom insisted with her often futile and argumentative 20/20 hindsight.

"There was no reason to take it off," Michelle rebutted. Thinking back to that time, I remember people having suggested she remove the second breast, but who knew the cancer would strike again?

As it would turn out, it was our genetic makeup that had already decided breast cancer would attack our family for generations to come.

When Michelle and my parents had returned to UCSF, my mom was asked if our family is Jewish; specifically Ashkenazi from Eastern European descent.

What does that matter, asked my mother.

As it turns out, she was told, there is a strong possibility that descendants of Ashkenazi Jews will have the BRCA genetic mutation.

Ashkenazi Jewish descendants have the highest prevalence of BRCA mutations of any population. That's what I read from a website called FORCE: an acronym for Facing Our Risk of Cancer Empowered. That website focuses on fighting hereditary breast and ovarian cancers. Members of this population are given a 1-in-40 chance of testing BRCA positive. It's this mutation that gives these Jews (and some other focused populations) a significantly higher chance of getting certain cancers such as breast and ovarian cancers, along with a few extras added to the list for women and men: melanoma and cancers that strike the colon, stomach, prostate and male breasts.

Mom began telling people, "Hitler won." Even though he didn't succeed in killing off all the Jews in Europe, after thinning out the Jewish gene pool, the bastard is still killing off the Jews, she would say.

Along with mom's revelation, now more than ever, she was extremely happy I married a Methodist man from Scottish descent instead of a Jewish man. In marrying Mark, I managed to reinforce our gene pool with the blue blood of Scottish kings and other colorful characters directly traced back to Charlemagne. (Both my father-in-law and Mark's brother had conducted many years of diligent detective work to detail the family tree) Without realizing, I'd secured somewhat of a safer future for my children. Or so I thought.

It was explained to me later, everyone has the BRCA gene. If it is mutated, your body is unable to fight off any breast, ovarian, or a selection of other nasty cancer cells that may form in your body.

Because Michelle had a bone marrow transplant which essentially kills you before they bring your insides back to life, there should have been no chance of her getting the breast cancer again. Her second round of breast cancer was an entirely new cancer, unrelated to her first experience. My parents were told by the doctors, it shouldn't have happened.

In the months that followed her treatments, my sister and parents were tested for the genetic mutation. Moreover, mom was told by UCSF, after Michelle's new diagnosis, they would be sending out letters of warning to other women who had received a bone marrow transplant. She said UCSF would tell women to get checked; their cancer may return if they test positive for the BRCA1 or BRCA2 genetic mutations.

Mom's test returned negative. Dad's test returned positive for BRCA1, as did Michelle's.

It makes sense, really, when you consider dad's mother and sister both died from breast cancer at young ages: dad said my grandmother was in her 40s and my aunt was 32.

Technically, dad's mother died from colon cancer; another target of the BRCA mutation. Regardless, dad told me how she had been treated for breast cancer, but ultimately, it was the cancer that spread to her colon that killed her. Ever since then, our family just says, she died from breast cancer.

Dad's niece (his sister's daughter) also tested positive and became a breast cancer survivor after having gone through treatments at the same time my sister was going through hers back in the mid-1990s.

It became my mom's mission to convince me to have the genetic test.

Actually, she had started learning about the genetic testing and what some had begun calling the "breast cancer gene" years before, shortly after Michelle's first round of cancer. She thought I should get tested, but I had resisted the idea for many years.

"If there's nothing I can do about it, I don't want to know. What's the point," I used to tell her. "If the test returns as positive, I'd just feel like a cancer time bomb. And anyway, if my health insurance found out, I'd never be able to get any coverage." How sad is that? Once again, health insurance was a key factor in our family's cancer story.

Also, I figured, how likely was it that I would get it if my sister already got it? Stupid, I know, but I honestly didn't want to know.

But now, facing Michelle's new cancer, my resolve weakened; I knew it was as though someone was hitting me over the head with the obvious. Regardless, there were several reasonable answers why I shouldn't find out.

I had put up blinders for years just so I didn't have to face the truth. I didn't want this information swimming around in my "what if" brain allowing my mind to slip into depression.

"If it were me, I'd want to know," my sister would tell me. "You'll be better prepared if you know."

"I already give myself regular exams," I said. That was mostly true; like many women, I did this when I remembered to do it, and I wasn't on any real schedule. "And since you had cancer the first time, I've been getting annual mammograms since I was 30. I'm doing what I need to do, so what else would change?"

Little did I know.

Eventually, I agreed to talk with the genetic counselor. By May, I had an appointment set up with Beth Crawford at UCSF on the same day my sister had one of her many surgeries.

Over the course of eight hours on the other side of the hospital, surgeons were working on Michelle to remove her second breast and ovaries.

While my sister was on the table, my parents came along with me to meet with Beth. She assured me, I was protected not only under federal law, but also by a more strict California law against any health insurance discrimination should I test positive for the genetic mutation. She told my parents, my concerns about health insurance were particularly common among people considering the test.

With the insurance issue resolved, my mother's response was blunt; I would expect nothing less.

"Now, will you take the fucking test?" mom demanded.

I agreed, my blood was drawn, boxed up and sent to a company back east; the only company in the country that does the testing because apparently, they hold the rights to the test.

I didn't know it then, but during the next year and a half, my mom would be making that long drive into the city with me to most of my appointments.

CHAPTER 3:
JUST KEEP BUSY

I'm not one who can wait patiently for test results. After my blood was sent off to some far away lab that held the key to my future in a vial, I was glad to be busy in my job at the school.

That school year, I had been teaching an art enrichment program at my children's school; one that would be closing because of dropping enrollment in our district and deep budget cuts.

If there was something good that came out of the school's bad situation, it was my job teaching the art program.

Even though many months passed when we didn't know if our school or another campus in the district would be shut down, the principal encouraged the school's PTA to use its funds on the students with extra programs, field trips, assemblies and a huge end-of-the-year party.

I got hired to teach one of those extras: the "Meet the Masters" art enrichment program. I took a very basic curriculum and expanded it into a course the children loved.

It felt great every time one of the students would drag their parents to my classroom so they could show all the art in the room. I had completely covered the walls with artwork stretching up onto the ceiling. That was a big change from the former art teacher who had a few posters on the walls and left the room mostly bare.

What was the point in that? I saw the walls, ceiling, even the front door, as a canvas. I used up every inch that I could to make art exciting for the children. If lack of funds prevented me from taking them to any of the several art museums in San Francisco, I did what I could to bring the museums' art to the students.

The teachers told me they liked how I taught the program.

Although, there were a couple who couldn't manage the noise factor in my classroom.

"Do you really want the class this loud?" one teacher asked.

"Sure, why not?" Art isn't meant to be restrained, I told her. The art room should be a safe place to go a little crazy; a haven where youngsters can express themselves and reveal their creativity.

Some teachers would get upset if the children didn't follow the directions precisely. They would get all fussy if they drew in the opposite direction as the example I showed them. One teacher, in particular, would shuffle the children out of my classroom as quickly as she could. I guess she thought I was teaching bad habits.

I'd been raised by an artist mother who rarely drew inside the lines in art and life, and there was always music. I incorporated music into my assemblies and in the classroom, adding to the general noise.

Most teachers enjoyed visiting my classroom and the biggest compliment came when I was teaching the kids about Claude Monet. Some teachers offered to pay me for the garden scene I had created in one corner of the room. They wanted to hang it in their classrooms the following year.

I created a scene out of Monet's water lily paintings; it was my interpretation of his familiar bridge, purple iris plants and a variety of blooms and lily pads.

The 3-D scene took on the feel of a popup book and included a Willow tree with branches and long strands of leaves hanging down from the ceiling. The children enjoyed sitting under the tree when they wanted to look at art books or when we gathered to review what they learned about a particular artist.

All my hard work seemed to pay off. It was wonderful to hear parents tell me how their child told them stories about Leonardo Da Vinci's inventions, or how they get excited when they saw Piet Mondrian's geometric designs carried over into modern advertising and architecture.

Thanks to my mom's experience at the San Francisco Art Institute where she had earned her bachelor's degree, I followed her advice about how to make the class interesting and entertaining for the children; tell vignettes from the artists' lives, she had told me, and the children will remember more of the lesson. I expanded the artist assemblies to include interesting details about what was happening in the world at the time each artist was alive. I brought in music from the period and made my own videos showing the art.

I learned how teaching could be so rewarding and loved what I was doing. Years later, children who had my class would continue to tell me how much they enjoyed my art program.

By the time the school's open house evening came along near the end of the school year, one of my close friends helped me transform the school's large auditorium into an art gallery to display the children's work.

It took us several days to get everything set up and the many hours of work kept my mind off of the nagging realities pressing down on my life.

After battling the school board throughout the year and adding my two cents at multiple public meetings on the matter of school closures, the district decided to eliminate our school; one that had secured a reputation as a top school in the district. It was frustrating and made no sense.

Nevertheless, there was still work to be done, and more ways to avoid my sister's breast cancer reality. That sounds so callous and heartless, but I had my specific role in her recovery. I was her sounding board and sanctuary where she could vent about how crappy life can be. It was mom's role to go with her to appointments.

By May, Michelle had completed all the chemo they would give her. At one point, they were forced to stop feeding the chemicals into her body because it nearly triggered a heart attack. During her first time with the cancer, they had given her such strong doses of chemo, her body couldn't withstand much more this second time.

They had to find safer chemo drugs; that meant giving her treatment that was significantly more expensive.

Anyone who has had cancer knows it is a costly process. Many times, health insurance may not cover medications that are not the generic versions of the drug.

My family has many stories of standing in line for medications and hearing the common discussion that the cancer patient's insurance won't cover a medication; the insurance will only cover a generic form, but the drug companies don't offer the drug as generic, thereby forcing the patients to make up the difference.

The patient, appearing weak and beaten by the disease, tells the pharmacist they can't pay for the drugs that help keep them alive. There's nothing the pharmacist can do, and the patient is left without the necessary drugs. It's as though it's the intention of the insurance companies to kill off their weakest clients who may not have the strength to work and earn the necessary money to pay for the life-saving drugs.

I'm proud of my parents and their empathy and generosity. Several times, when they have waited in these lines, they came to the rescue of desperate patients and paid for their life-saving medication.

As summer neared, Michelle's surgeons implanted an expander in her chest to start recreating her breast's shape. The expander, slowly filled with saline at weekly appointments, is used to stretch the skin before a breast implant can be installed.

Unfortunately, within a week of the expander's installation, Michelle began experiencing intensified pain in the area of the foreign object. An infection had developed. The expander would have to be removed.

Complicating matters, she was experiencing a separate pain caused by her gall bladder; that organ had to be cut out of her body before the expander could be extracted from her breast.

Her health insurance wouldn't allow UCSF to remove the gall bladder because it was unassociated with her cancer. Therefore, Michelle was transferred from UCSF to the VA hospital for the removal of her gall bladder and to get her infection and pain under control before sending her back to UCSF to remove the expander.

One afternoon during this complicated process, I visited the VA to see my sister and check on mom to see if she, too, was holding it together. After hanging out with Michelle for a bit, mom asked me to take a little walk down the hall with her. Arm in arm, we strolled down the quiet corridor. Mom was upset. Tears began flowing as she spoke in hushed tones.

"What's going on? What did the doctor say?" I asked.

"Oh, Joey. Your sister is in so much pain. They've been giving her so much medicine trying to get rid of the pain and the infection, but nothing is working. The doctor told me, because she has had to take so many medicines, if this antibiotic doesn't work, there's nothing else they can give her. She could die from the staph infection," she spoke through tears.

"Oh, mom," I pulled her close for a hug.

"This is the strongest drug they've got, Joey."

What can you do in this situation? Hearing this news would

15

leave anyone feeling impotent. If the antibiotics didn't work, my sister's health could be fixed only if her body successfully attacked and killed this infection that did what it could to rip away another child's life from my parents.

Mom didn't want Michelle to worry about what would happen if this medicine didn't work; there was no point in telling her about the doctor's warning.

Later, Michelle told me, at the time, she didn't care about anything happening around her because they had given her a bed that had air pumped into it, adjusting to her body any time she would move. The comfort offered by the bed coupled with the pain medicine helped lessen her discomfort, if even only for a week.

Thankfully, the medicine took hold and Michelle pulled through before being transferred back to UCSF for another surgery. Once again, she was left with half a flat chest.

As she healed, the disfigured skin of her butchered breast remained exceedingly sensitive to anything it came in contact with. Repeatedly, she tugged her shirt away from her skin. I noticed her posture became slightly hunched over to account for the extra-sensitive skin.

Several months would pass before her surgeon replaced the expander in her breast. Meanwhile, because her immune system was so thrashed, she remained susceptible to illness and had to be careful to avoid anyone who was sick.

That meant, while mom and I were able to talk her out of attending our cousin's wedding where she would be around crowds of people, she took a big chance attending Jesse's fifth grade graduation ceremony and being among throngs of children. There was no way she was going to skip her favorite nephew's graduation.

In preparation of Jesse's commencement, shortly before the end of the school year, I was asked by the graduation committee if I would paint backdrops for the stage. My longtime friend Harmony purchased white sheets to stretch into canvases on stand-alone frames.

Painting these canvases took more than a week up on that stage in the school's auditorium. Staying with a Hawaiian theme, on one side I painted a tropical beach in front of mountains covered in lush jungle. On the other sheet canvas, I painted a jumbo wave with a surfer crouched down and enjoying his ride inside the glassy structure.

During lunchtime, the children got excited to see the progress of the paintings. They would ask questions, or just watch me paint.

I remained busy with the art program and backdrop painting project leading up to that last day of school. My work provided a reasonable excuse to my family about why I couldn't be with them for this evening or that day. I felt guilty for avoiding Michelle's reality, and still do. Yet, I couldn't spend too much time with my sister. I hate to admit it, but this was my way of handling the foul situation.

After Renee had been killed, my natural shyness transformed into the depths of introversion. And after Michelle got cancer the first time and we all thought she would die after the doctor gave her six months to live, I began sinking back into that shy world.

I couldn't bear losing another sister. During Michelle's first bout with cancer, I kept busy at my job as a newspaper reporter to avoid the reality my parents—mostly mom—was left to deal with.

I don't think my family understood how much Michelle's life-threatening disease impacted me. I was snapping at everyone and everything.

One night at work, I got into my first quarrel with my editor about a story. I thought it should be given a better position than he offered. It should be on the front page, as opposed to this other writer's story that had nothing to do with the paper's audience or the cities we wrote about.

This writer—about 15 years older than I—was new to the paper and conducted herself like a snake in the grass. Every chance she got, she was a back-stabbing, two-faced bitch. For some reason, my editor couldn't see it. And the crazy thing is, there was no reason to act that way. The people at this paper tended to be particularly supportive of each other and worked well as a team. I welcomed her as another writer on the paper, but she was singularly underhanded and devious in her actions.

I was in the middle of an argument about my story when the phone rang. He and I were still arguing when I realized it was my mom on the line.

"Joey, your sister tried to commit suicide," my mom cried.

"Is she okay?"

She told me how she and my sister had gotten into another fight and Michelle tried to swallow a handful of pills; not the kind that would have killed her, but mom didn't know that at the time.

My parents felt compelled to call the police because Michelle was acting so irrationally.

After Michelle had finished chemotherapy, the doctors took her off of a cocktail of drugs that were meant to help keep her calm and relieve anxiety during the process; drugs such as Ativan, Paxil and Zofran. When she went cold turkey off the medications, mom said, "She went bonkers." She described her as hyper and a nervous wreck. She should have been taken off the drugs slowly to help prevent the erratic behavior that lead to her suicide attempt and her aggressive reaction to the police showing up at my parent's home.

Because of her surgeries, Michelle can no longer put her arms behind her back without suffering immense pain. The cops were brutal with her as they handcuffed her behind her back. They ignored my parent's pleas to stop their actions because they were injuring her.

"I'm on my way, mom," I told her and ended the call.

"What's wrong?" my editor asked.

"My sister tried to kill herself." Our argument was over. "You know what? Do whatever the hell you want with the story. I don't give a shit."

"I hope she's okay," he said with sincerity.

Through my concern and shock about my sister, I was a bit bitchy when I responded. "Yeah. Thanks." I left.

During her first breast cancer, and now during her second round, it was my parents who went to the doctor appointments with Michelle. Of course, this time around, the chemo and treatments didn't deplete my sister of any of her hyper energy as was the case a decade before. Making matters worse, every time she had to go to the doctor, she would become unglued. After what she had experienced during the first cancer, her reaction was understandable.

This time, there were fights and phone calls every time friction built because my older sister didn't want to follow my parent's advice or demands. This time, Michelle maintained her hyper personality and generally put up a fight.

That's where my participation came into play. Again, it's not that I wasn't involved in her recovery; as I mentioned earlier, I served a specific role for Michelle. I was a sounding board for her and mom every time they had a fight. I helped them cool down or find some middle ground. Mark would suggest I begin charging for my services. I should have become a shrink, he said.

"Will you tell your sister she's being a horse's ass," mom would demand on the phone after I said hello. "She won't listen to me or your father, and she's going to get killed. The doctor said she's crazy and she shouldn't do this. I'm tired of fighting with her. Will you please explain this to her?"

It didn't matter what the issue was. That was a very common call. But Michelle is a grown woman. She was going to do what she wanted, regardless of how her decisions impacted anyone around her.

Whatever the issue, it became my job to mediate and quell their clashes until the next time. In the process, I hoped I wouldn't be slammed by either side.

If I displayed too much support for mom, my sister would rev up in her own idiosyncratic hyper talk that gets louder and louder. There's no way to get a word in edgewise, and before you know it, she's just screaming in your ear like nails on a chalkboard. All you want her to do is shut up.

"Well, Joe," she'd yell in her snarky, bitchy manner. "If I do what mom and dad want then...." It didn't matter what anyone said; generally, she would do whatever the hell she wanted, and fuck everyone else, no matter the consequences. Then, everyone around her was left to clean up after her calamities.

Once in a while, if I used every ounce of energy to keep my voice low and calm as though I was in a gorilla cage trying to avoid being the target of a shit-tossing war, I might convince her to slow down, take a breath, step back, listen to my reality check and stop jumping into the fire. If I couldn't get her to withdraw her impulsive reaction and she did what she wanted, too many times my parents would consider it my fault that I didn't stop her. That's not the best incentive to try again, but I did; I did it for my parents in an attempt to protect my sister whenever possible.

On the other hand, if I backed up my sister, mom would go off in a rage and there was no pulling her off the hyperbole ledge. I wouldn't hear the end of it until she finally dragged my father into the mess which got me into deeper shit. (Yeah, thanks, sis.)

"Will you talk to her?" my mom would yell at my dad.

Dad learned long ago, if he gets involved, eventually, Michelle and mom would gang up on him and me. Therefore, he tries his best to stay out of the repeated battles. Mom just considers this reality as being part of a typical dysfunctional American family.

When he did get pulled into the battles, it was with utter reluctance that dad would take the phone from my mother.

"Look, we're just worried about your sister," was the generic line. He would remain calm, unlike my mother who would stand glaring down at my father who just wanted to watch some TV. Mom's hands on her hips, her expression pinched and angry, and her head slightly cocked, she'd be huffing and snarling like a bull waiting for my dad to say the wrong thing. Then she would start yelling at him, too.

"What? I said what you wanted," he'd respond as she'd yank the phone away from him.

"Why are you saying that? You don't know what the hell you're talking about," she'd respond.

"Then don't give me the goddamn phone if all you're going to do is yell at me. That's why I don't want to get mixed up in all her crap. She does this to us every time," dad would respond and then their fight would escalate.

When we were children and hated each other's guts, Michelle and I knew, as soon as our parents began their fight, we could return to playing or watching TV.

I'm used to the general battles, but one of the worst phone calls I can get is when my dad rings me and quietly declares, "You know, you really hurt your mother."

Those few words are enough to cut through my heart when my dad says that to me. Ugh! That's true power. I wish my mom would figure that one out; she doesn't have to be loud and yell to produce a desired impact. But after all, she came from the "wait until your father gets home" generation. Consequently, she always lost battles.

I know my mom doesn't think I did anything either time Michelle was dealing with her cancer, but it was me who would promise to talk to Michelle when my parents no longer could get through to her. It was my job to calm my sister through her crying and anger fits and offer some reasoning and a practical plan.

And when mom's energy and patience as caretaker would dwindle, every so often I would be attacked for my lack of providing any cancer-elimination participation. That's when I would be the recipient of mom's "You're a terrible daughter/sister" rants.

Before I go on, I know my mother is going to read this. This is where she's going to call me and insist I made her out to be a horrible mother. Mom, you know (as do I) the opposite is true. You are a saint to put up with all the terrible news and fight through trials of life as well as you have. There's no one else I'd rather call when I need help because you are the advocate I want in my corner when the shit hits the proverbial fan. But everyone has their moments, and no one is perfect, right? So calm down and read on.

Regardless of my poor level of participation in Michelle's physical recovery, after our mother's attacks, my sister would reveal a kinder side and tell me how vital our conversations and phone calls were.

When she needed someone to talk to, it didn't matter what it was; I would listen to her rattle on about our parents, the doctors, treatments, her loneliness, her future, the pain she was in, or whatever. She told me that's what she needed most from me. Therefore, that's what I gave her.

I'm glad I could offer her at least that. I'll always feel guilty for not doing more.

CHAPTER 4:
THE SUMMER BEFORE THE STORM

Shortly after Jesse graduated from fifth grade and right before Mark and I were going to take the kids on a cruise with a little extra money we had, my dad had a stroke.

My 78-year-old "sweet tooth" father wasn't very good about caring for his diabetes over the years, and the side effects became increasingly severe as he got older. This time, he ended up lying on a hospital bed at Kaiser, smelling of urine and having difficulty using his left arm and hand.

For a few years, dad's health had been deteriorating noticeably; he had to have open-heart surgery, skin cancer treatments, eye surgeries and other treatments in response to various issues. But it was this stroke that served as a turning point in his life.

Suddenly, my father had transformed into an old man. His physical limitations added to my mother's growing frustration and anger at my dad for not having taken better care of himself. She wanted to travel in their retirement, not be tied down to medical obligations. Unless she welded a boat to her minivan, the only place she would be cruising to on a regular basis was dad's many doctors' offices.

More complications surfaced because of the medications necessary for dad's recovery. If he took the appropriate medicine, it would damage his kidneys. If he didn't take the medication, he could get a blood clot that would stop his heart or lead to a stroke.

The doctors stepped back and took a wait-and-see approach, and we all remained vigilant.

Dad did pull through, but not without first having to spend some time in a rehabilitation facility before returning home to face the wrath of my mother's mood swings.

As well, this was the first time dad's mind seemed to be impacted by the disease, but mom wasn't ready to deal with that yet.

She didn't want to face the fact that the stroke may have impacted my father's "Atticus Finch" logical mind. Her denial and his difficulties served as the catalyst for a series of battles that summer. When he monitored his own medications, dad would take the wrong amount or simply forget to take his meds (including insulin). This would start a fight that generally resulted in mom calling me to complain about how dad doesn't do anything to care for his own body.

When she tried to help him with the doses, dad would snap at mom because he was accustomed to being in control of his medications. They would have to find some common ground allowing mom to keep her husband alive, and dad to maintain some control.

"Mom, after the stroke, I don't think he realizes what he's doing. I think it changed him; his mind," I told her.

"But Joey, it's so damn frustrating. I've become his fucking caretaker." She gave example after example of what he was doing. It wasn't that she didn't love him; this transition was extraordinarily difficult and frustrating and exhausting. And I knew my mother hated seeing her beloved husband struggling to keep control over his mind and body as he aged. Revealing her frustration, she said, "I'm just so pissed at your father. He did this to himself, and now, he's dragging me down with him."

She was right, to a point, but I had to remind her, "Mom, you should know by now, diabetes is a progressive disease. Yes, he shouldn't have been sneaking bits of candy, and eating stuff he wasn't supposed to consume; but this is one of those odd diseases because you don't always see the effects of it. That is unless you don't take your medicine."

I reminded her of an elderly woman I had interviewed for a story. She was fit, watched her diet, and one day she decided she would be fine without the medicine. She stopped taking her insulin, her husband had told me. I had spoken with her only a few weeks prior to her death and ironically, we had been talking about diabetes and how it's a hidden disease.

"Next thing I know, the woman slips into a coma and dies. You don't want that to happen to dad, right?"

"No, I know, but…," mom started.

"Dad's been dealing with this disease for decades, and now it's catching up with him. So, cut him some slack. Yes, you are going to have to keep a watchful eye and make sure he takes the correct amount of insulin because—and I know this is going to be difficult to hear—I believe the stroke impacted his mind. I don't think he can do these things on his own now; at least, not yet. And to get mad at him for it is like kicking a 3-legged dog because they walk with a limp."

"Yeah. I know you're right, but…," I didn't let her finish.

"No buts. You chose to marry a man seven years your senior. Think about what I'm going to face when Mark gets old and decrepit. He's a decade older than me," I tried distracting her attention away from dad and lightening her mood.

"Oh, you really *are* screwed. What are you going to do when he gets old and he can't wipe his ass?"

"I've already told him, there's no way I'm going to wipe his ass. If I have to do that, I'll end up puking on him."

"Eeew," my mom laughed. "But you wiped your children's asses. Why won't you wipe your husband's ass?"

"They were babies. That's different. And it was disgusting then, too. I don't deal well with adult bodily fluids. It's like that joke about how a New Yorker responds to someone who has collapsed and requires resuscitation. You better start breathing or ya gonna fuckin' die!"

"Oh, you really are a bitch," mom laughed.

"You know it. All I keep hearing is my dead Southern mother-in-law's voice that time when she was describing one of her neighbors who was always getting yelled at by his wife. 'That poor man,'" I mimicked her Southern drawl.

Because of my dad's health and mom going generally crazy having to care for him and help my sister with her cancer, we had offered to cancel our trip to stay home and help, but by the time dad was moved into rehab, my parents encouraged us to go. There was nothing more we could do, they said, before dad added some playful Jewish guilt, "That's okay. Go have some fun while I'm stuck here with your mother. Don't worry about us."

We flew to Texas where Mark and I took the kids on a Carnival cruise out of Galveston. This was the perfect escape from reality for our family. Our excitement grew as stresses dissolved with each step forward up the gangplank. Every passenger is given a card which opens their room, serves as a credit card for purchases made onboard, and to use as their identification card at every port.

Stepping through the gangway, one by one, our cards were inserted into a machine that sounds a unique "dang" when your identity is confirmed. And with that wonderful chime of approval, we were allowed to enter Carnival's gilded fantasy world. The kids were excited, giggling and expressing wide-eyed glee as we wound our way through corridors and found our stateroom. From there, we began exploring the ship and made our way up to the top of the vessel to look out as we sailed away on silky waters to Grand Cayman, Jamaica and Cozumel.

Other than the non-stop buffet on board the ship, our favorite stop far from reality was Grand Cayman where we got to swim with the sting rays, sail across the most beautiful, clear blue water, and do some "power shopping."

Yes, after returning from a day of sailing, snorkeling and kissing a stingray to attract seven years good luck, in my quest for tanzanite during the limited time before the ship would leave, I rushed my family from one amazing jewelry store to the next.

Within a 90-minute period, I managed to lead them through more than 10 jewelry shops. When time is limited, mom had taught me how to scan quickly through jewelry cases. "Nope. It's not here," I'd tell my family. They would race to catch up with me as I left for the next store.

Periodically, we would slow our pace while Mark enjoyed being treated like a rich American when we were taken into the back rooms where the "good stuff" was located; incredible pieces we couldn't afford, but they were fun to try on. Another thing mom taught me; never feel intimidated to ask.

"They're a merchant. A sale is money in their pocket, no matter who buys their product," mom would tell me.

And it didn't matter that we were in shorts and T-shirts. Some of my dad's richest, multimillionaire clients wore modest clothes and didn't put on airs of superiority.

I've passed on these lessons to my own children. As dad always said, "Rich or poor, people put their pants on one leg at a time like everyone else."

It was fun to feel glamorous for a while, trying on necklaces dripping with diamonds and tanzanite. Mark enjoyed studying the historical jewelry made from centuries-old gold coins once carried by pirates and royal navy ships.

It fills me with joy to see the world's stresses slip away from my family's shoulders, if only for a week. The pure happiness in my silly daughter's face lights up any scene. And my son's "Mona Lisa" smile reveals his warmth of spirit and zeal for adventure.

When I was growing up, I remember families in which the parents would go traveling the world, but they would leave their children at home. My parents wanted us to experience different places and cultures, therefore they took us along on most of their travels; I've done the same for our children.

Perhaps they won't experience too much cultural variety visiting a tropical island like Grand Cayman, but certainly, they saw a glimpse of the outside world when we visited Jamaica.

We hired a taxi driver, Steadman, to take us around at Montego Bay. We didn't take a tour. My parents rarely took tours in the many places they have traveled.

"Just hire a taxi and let them show you around. You'll see more than if you take a tour," my mom always reminds us before we head off on an adventure.

My parents learned to do that when they lived overseas while dad was in the Air Force. He was stationed in places including North Africa and Spain. My eldest sister, Renee, was born in Madrid before Michelle was born in Michigan. The latter isn't as romantic as being born in Spain, but getting booted out of Europe and sent to snowbound Michigan is what happens when an officer's wife—my mom—slaps a colonel after he made a pass at her by placing his hand on her ass.

My parents have journeyed all over the world, and they enjoy taking the roads less traveled to explore new towns and places. They taught that to me and my sisters.

Steadman took us to a hotel by the beach that offered waterslides at the pool and one of those meandering lazy rivers on which we could float and find cool relief from the tropical heat. Many hotels in the area were protected by guards and high fences designed to prevent the outside dangers of the city from infringing on the sheltered fantasy world created within its walls. This hotel was no different.

The kids were excited to go down the water slides that were

several stories tall. But when Sophie nearly drowned, we quickly realized, the pool at the bottom of the slide wasn't governed like American safety standards. The drop at the slide's finish landed in the pool's deep end. Moreover, the water rushed down the slides with such force, the quick current resulted in the swimmer being held down under the water.

Mark and I remained near the base of the slide because Sophie wasn't a strong swimmer, but it was difficult to extract her from the current. This caused some panic until we finally grabbed her and she surfaced while coughing and choking on water. The experience left her apprehensive to go down the slide unless Mark or I doubled with her.

After lunch, Steadman drove us up into the hills and to another hotel with spectacular views overlooking Montego Bay. Again, the hotel was gated. It had the feeling of a fort protected by a strong vantage point high up on the side of that hill.

It wasn't until we traveled down from the peak when the impoverished city began closing in on us. Our children got their first taste of what a Third World Country looks like.

We drove along narrow streets where the buildings were crumbling as though they'd been bombed or abandoned as unrecoverable remnants of an earthquake. The sidewalks were crowded with locals wearing worn-out clothing juxtaposed against groups of youngsters adorned in required uniforms for school.

Concern washed over our children's faces as they looked out through the tinted windows of Steadman's air-conditioned van. People stared at our slowly passing vehicle or carried on with their day. It was the first time Jesse and Sophie had seen such magnified poverty; they remained silent and periodically glanced at me or Mark.

If I'm being honest, I suppose I'd have to say, I wondered why he took us through that part of town. Was it to prove a point? To remind the Americans of how miserable life can be?

I am so very glad to have been raised in America. I appreciate what I have, but everything is relative, and I don't consider myself rich.

Did these people have what appeared to be shitty lives? We assumed they had less than we did, but again, everything is relative. I'm thankful we don't live in a hut, but we live in California, after all; a state considered one of the most expensive places to live in the

United States.

People we know who live elsewhere in our country don't comprehend why we laugh when they say they can buy a house for $50,000. In Marin or many parts of the wine country where we live, you can't buy a garage for that amount of money. Therefore, generally it's a struggle to live here and we have been trying to move away for a while.

Sitting there in that van and looking out at the poor conditions in that Jamaican city, I must admit, I did glance over to make sure the doors were locked. Not that locked car doors would deter anyone who was determined to get in.

It wasn't uncommon for tourists to be attacked in Jamaica. Not long before our trip, a busload of tourists was ambushed during a planned cruise tour to a plantation; it was one of those tours people think are the safest choice because the cruise lines sell them.

Still, I would lock my car doors in areas of town within 10 miles of where we live. Likewise, I remember a trip to New York when I was a teenager when my dad wanted to show us his old neighborhood in the Bronx. Looking around at dad's shattered community, I can still see my mother's troubled expression and hear dad saying, "Roll 'em up and lock 'em up." We didn't stay very long.

Use a little common sense and you can travel safely to most places. This is what my parents taught me.

"Mommy, why are their buildings broken?" my daughter whispered her question with furrowed brow.

"This is how a lot of people around the world live, sweetie," I told my 7-year-old. She looked out the windows and tried to understand.

By the time we made our way back to the cruise ship and had said our goodbyes to Steadman, the children appeared exceedingly happy and appreciative to be back in the pristine world of Carnival.

I would go on cruises every year, if we could afford it. You see, I hate to cook. Having a menu placed in front of me at every meal is heaven; that, and finding my little home on the sea cleaned every day and never having to lift a finger. Spending time with the family and visiting new places are the bonuses when the remainder of your life is filled with the mundane.

All too soon, we found ourselves having to return home to our daily grind. It didn't take long for the kids to complain of their boredom from sitting around the house that summer.

Jesse remained busy in the afternoons with swimming. That summer, he had joined the local swim team and we became a swim family.

Soon enough, it was time for Jesse's first swim meet; his team's biggest meet of the year.

It was the end of July when we all awakened at 6 a.m. and rushed to head out the door. We were going to the Redwood Empire Swim League meet (or RESLs, as the team calls it) in El Cerrito over in the East Bay.

On the first day of the meet, my parents left a while after Jesse's first of two races. Thankfully, they took Michelle home with them; she'd been acting like a stage mom, getting in the way of the coaches at their tent by the pool when they would talk to Jesse before his event.

At one point, Mark and I watched from across the pool as she went so far as to crouch alongside Jesse's two kneeling coaches. They had been talking to him as he floated in the water holding onto the pool's cement edge after taking a break from warming up for his event.

"What the hell is she doing?" I said to my husband as we watched her trying to look important and impressive. Some of the coaches repeatedly asked her to leave their area.

"Yeah, she was doing what *they* did and looking at me with this creepy look," my son told me later, detailing the frustrating, uncomfortable scene.

"I just wanted to make sure they were giving him good advice and telling him everything he needed to know," was her response when I confronted her on her actions.

"Like you would know what to tell him? Michelle, when were you ever on a swim team?" I asked. She paused for a moment.

"Okay, yeah, you're right. But I just wanted to make sure...."

"Michelle, they are good coaches. Let them do their work."

"I'm just so excited for him."

I knew she was proud of him; as did Jesse. Even when she lives far away, she still tries to remain a very active and generous aunt in my children's lives, and I greatly appreciate her participation. She adores them and loves spending time with them.

It's just that, at Jesse's first big sports contest, I didn't want my sister getting in the way of him enjoying the experience and the team. But she couldn't resist offering advice on a sport she knew little about. She only created conflict with the people who were there to help my son improve his skills as a swimmer.

It never sinks in that once she leaves and returns to her life somewhere else, it is the rest of us who must deal with the residue of her demanding personality and abrasive nature.

When my parents said they were thinking of leaving the meet that day, I was happy to hear this news that would release us from the added stress of Michelle's presence.

As they were packing up their chairs, Sophie decided she wanted to accompany her bubby (bubby is a pet name for grandma) and papa to swim in their pool and sleep over at their house. Unfortunately, her spontaneity created an open seat in our car for the drive home.

"Then how about I stay and drive home with you guys," Michelle asked with zeal. My insides tightened.

"No," Mark and I simultaneously exclaimed, before looking at each other with sudden panic. *Please mom, don't back up Michelle like you always do. Please mom.*

"But you could help me with Sophie," added mom. *Phew.* Lucky for us, mom wanted Michelle to share the responsibility of watching and playing with our daughter.

"Oh," Michelle sounded disappointed. Mark could tell I felt a little ashamed for excluding my sister's participation and gave me his "don't change your mind now" expression. "I guess you don't want to drive back to our house tonight," she added.

"Well, not if Sophie is spending the night," Mark said, adding more excuses about being too tired at the end of the long day.

I felt guilty about the way things played out. And yet, I wanted to eliminate my family's single-minded focus on how Jesse placed in his races. Who gives a shit? I was just glad he jumped in the pool with hundreds of people watching. It's intimidating the first time you line up to race. I knew what that felt like because I had been on my high school's swim team. I was proud of my 11-year-old son's participation, especially after the fears he expressed earlier in the day.

While making our way through town to the swim center that morning, Jesse said he had changed his mind and suddenly didn't want to compete.

"We managed to talk him into trying. I don't want him to hear anything but positive feedback from his family," I stressed to my sister when I saw her at the pool that morning. Being a new swimmer on the team, there was plenty he needed to learn and improve; he knew this and didn't need to hear about it from his family. "Just let him have fun with it so he'll stick with the sport."

"Yeah, you're right," she said. But she couldn't resist.

Jesse's first event was the 50 freestyle (two laps of the pool). Just like many other young, inexperienced swimmers, he wasn't comfortable diving off the block or doing a flip turn off the wall. Naturally, those two elements slowed his time and left him at a disadvantage against the experienced swimmers.

Instead of diving off the block, he sprang off the cement deck in leap-frog fashion, making a large splash as he hit the water. After regaining his composure, he stroked his way toward the other end of the pool. Instead of a smooth flip turn, he grabbed the wall and lifted his head to suck in some air. He looked up at me and Mark standing at the end of his lane before pushing off the wall and heading for the finish.

After the race, my "expert" sister wasted little time to point out his flaws when he came over to us.

He was smiling shyly when he arrived. He looked up at us waiting for our response.

"We're so proud of you, little bug! You did so well," I said as I wrapped my arms around his bare back and pulled him close for a huge hug. He returned my embrace while Mark patted his back and repeated the praises.

"Mommy, you're getting wet." He was concerned the pool water dripping off him was soaking my clothes.

"I don't care about that. I'm just so proud of you. Did you have fun? Were you nervous?"

"I was nervous at first, but once I jumped in and started swimming, I was fine."

"You did so great," my sister started.

That's great, now stop saying anything. Please, just stop. Please....

"If you would just dive off the block and do the flip turns, you'd go even faster and you might win." She just had to say it. *Who gives a shit if he wins his first race?* I gave her a disapproving look and watched my son's excitement subside.

31

"We're not worried about that now," I said to my sister. And then to my son, "We're so proud of you, Jesse."

My parents congratulated him, but reinforced my sister's critique before he wandered off through the crowd to go talk to his coaches.

All I had to do was look at Michelle before she responded with regret. "I did a mom, didn't I?" She meant offering a compliment before ending with a criticism.

"Yup. I told you I wanted to keep it positive, but you just had to do it, didn't you?"

"Yeah, you're right," she said.

Sophie didn't want to stay, and dad was likely glad to get out of the sun when they gathered up all their belongings and left for the day.

The next morning, after leaving our warmer Sonoma County town and crossing over the Richmond-San Rafael Bridge toward El Cerrito for our second day of the meet, we weren't prepared for the chilly weather after having enjoyed high temperatures the prior day.

The low clouds never broke that day, and the wind picked up as the frigid morning slipped into a blustery afternoon. It was the middle of July and temperatures were in the mid-50s. My light sweatshirt barely provided any warmth and my flip-flops left my feet bare and increasingly numb.

Until they could escape the frigid scene, huddled under the team's canopies sat swimmers and parents bundled in long swim parkas and under fleece blankets. Hours passed as they waited for their races to start or their day to end.

"When I start feeling drowsy, I'll be freezing to death," I joked with Mark. Jesse and I bundled up under the two old towels we'd brought with us from home. Luckily, Mark (who wears shorts, no matter the season) had an extra jacket in his car for Jesse who hadn't brought a sweatshirt after it had been so hot the day before.

Jesse and I both complained to Mark, that had we taken my car instead of his hybrid equipped with no emergency kid supplies, not only would we have had blankets, extra towels and jackets, we'd also have had the hand warmers I keep in the back.

"Why do you have hand warmers?" he asked. "Why do you keep hand warmers in your car in July?"

"Mommy got them at REI," Jesse defended me.

"Yeah. In case the car breaks down on a cold night, or we're up in the snow or something," I said.

"But we don't live in the snow," Mark said. "And it's July."

"I realize that, but sometimes we go to the snow. And I don't want to end up like that family that took a wrong turn, and they all died during the snow storm."

"Whatever."

"Whatever? Screw whatever. I'm freezing!" I nagged.

Periodically, Jesse and I would make trips to the bathrooms that remained steamy from the steady stream of swimmers' taking hot showers after each race. I found myself crowding the hot-air hand-dryers mounted to the walls in the damp, women's bathroom. I would try to direct the hot air toward my feet that appeared to be turning deeper shades of red and blue with each passing hour.

Mark and I were thankful Sophie was still at my parent's home in sunny Marin. She wasn't with us freezing to death and whining about wanting to leave. We were also grateful for Jesse's inexperience as a swimmer.

Because his times were still slow, there was no chance he would qualify for the finals. Woohoo! That meant he was done by 1:30 p.m. that second day. We could go find someplace warm to enjoy a late lunch before heading over to the giant IKEA store nearby.

We wanted to find items to redecorate Jesse's room. Because he would be starting junior high in the fall, we didn't want him to feel uncomfortable about bringing any new friends to the house; his room was still decorated as a nursery with giraffe's and various characters from children's stories my mom painted before he was born.

Walking through the gigantic IKEA building was overwhelming. There's a steady flow of customers moving along the meandering pathways and it makes you feel like you have to keep moving forward. The people travel like schools of fish passing through themed rooms set up according to style.

If it were after closing time, it would make for a perfect scene out of a movie during which people get locked inside and pretend they have a different life than their own, all based on whatever design they entered.

We made up our own little sketches of life. There were small kitchens perfect for a studio apartment in San Francisco or New York City. We relaxed in our "new" living rooms, trying out couches we couldn't afford and watching the frozen scene on the fake flatscreen televisions mounted on the temporary store walls.

That's what IKEA is: playing "house" for adults. It's just a bigger playground.

Absent a solid plan, we left with few items for his room, but somehow managed to fill up our cart with odds and ends that we simply had to have. Jesse picked out a lamp, and we purchased an area rug for the kitchen.

We planned on returning with better focus and actual dimensions so that we could buy shelves and a proper desk to replace the garage sale desk I bought and painted with bright colors and his hand prints. I had seen something like it in a magazine with children's room designs and thought it would look cute in Jesse's room as a way to preserve his little paw prints.

Before several of my relatives had begun dying or downsizing and giving me the furniture they wanted to get rid of, I enjoyed finding furniture at garage sales and fixing them up for our home. Jesse's desk, a side table, a dresser, the coffee table; I would refinish them and recycle them into lovely, restored pieces.

But after my grandparents died, and later grandma's sister died, I ended up with tables, book shelves, a gargantuan television, cabinets, a gaudy, gilded bed frame and more furniture to fill up my home.

"You've got too much crap in your house." That's one of my mother's favorite comments when she visits.

"I can't help it if everyone keeps dying. It's everybody else's shit. It all ends up in my house," I responded.

"Why don't you get rid of some of it?" she asked. "Like that lamp. I always hated that lamp." Mom pointed to one of grandma's favorites; a garish table lamp that stands several feet high and sits on top of the black-stained side table that used to be in her home. Grandma liked Asian designs from Gump's in San Francisco.

I have a lot of grandma's black furniture; including a cabinet that mom wanted to get rid of.

"But I want that little cabinet," I told her. "It holds many happy memories." Grandma always kept special kid items in that sideboard. After my grandparents greeted us with warm hugs, it was the first place I'd head to when we arrived at their home. Sometimes, she'd add various puzzles and other games making it fun to see what she hid for us.

"Well, if you really want it. It's expensive furniture; I just don't like something so dark in my house." Mom prefers a casual, lighter style in her home.

I'm not a huge fan of dark furniture either, but periodically, I open that cabinet and the sound of the latch releasing takes me back to my grandmother's living room.

I can still feel the warm summer breeze flowing in from the patio through the sliding glass doors. I can hear my grandmother and mom chatting, sitting at the round wood table next to the kitchen.

Grandma would tell mom all the latest gossip about the family, or what she heard about someone mom went to school with at Lowell High School. She might tell about someone from the old neighborhood when they lived in the Marina in San Francisco where they owned "Arlene's" dry cleaning shop on Chestnut Street. They named it after my mom.

I envision my tan grandfather walking into the room wearing his bathing suit and asking if we kids want to go jump in the pool; or maybe he has discovered some new hobby.

Magic tricks, the concertina, sculpting class, writing stories from his childhood, the electric car he built out of the body of an old Toyota and would drive around Menlo Park. And every visit, he'd lead us into the kitchen where he had a treat drawer like other people keep a junk drawer.

"Want a sweet?" he'd ask as he took a See's dark-chocolate lollipop out of the drawer and removed the wrapper. He always had See's lollipops and other sweets squirreled away in that drawer and hidden in kitchen cabinets. There was always ice cream at my grandparent's home and an excess of food.

"Essin, mine kin," my grandma would say to me in Yiddish, meaning, "Eat, my child." I loved sleeping over at their house. They always took me out to eat when grandpa wasn't making his "bubbalas." A bubbala was some sort of omelet-like concoction that he would finish by sprinkling a heavy layer of sugar over the top.

If we were at their dry cleaning shop in Menlo Park, we would walk around the block to Alice's restaurant where my grandma said I could order anything I wanted. Generally, it was a grilled cheese and one of their jumbo milkshakes.

"Do you want another one," grandma would ask. "Anything you want, you can have. Essin, mine kin."

I miss my grandparents. I miss their hugs. I miss grandma's stories about when she was young, growing up in the Bronx. I miss grandpa's creative, young, adventurous spirit. I miss going shopping with grandma. She loved shopping, and she would have loved walking through IKEA, or clothes shopping with Sophie and touching everything.

Grandma was keenly sensitive to texture, and she passed that along to me. Walking through IKEA, I would drag my hand along a couch to feel the texture of the fabric, the smooth finish of the wood or the coolness of metal.

"Why do you touch everything as you walk by it," my son asked me once. I told him about my grandma and how she did the same thing; it was a way to test the quality of the product. Grandma said the quality was more important than the quantity. I was glad such a mundane act as going to the store could connect my children to my beloved grandparents. Jesse was only a toddler when grandma died, and grandpa followed not long after. I wish Sophie could have known them. She and my grandma would have gotten along famously.

CHAPTER 5:
BAD NEWS AND MORE BAD NEWS

For years, my mom had been bugging me to be tested to see if I carried the BRCA1 and/or BRCA2 genetic mutation. The day had finally arrived when I would find out the results of that test and its impact on my future.

Up to the very moment when I heard the results, I didn't want to know. I'm sure that sounds ridiculous and reckless, but I didn't want to live my life in fear of something that may never happen. When my sister was diagnosed with breast cancer the second time, I knew it would be stupid not to get tested, but sometimes ignorance really is bliss.

When my genetic counselor at UCSF called and said she wanted to fit me into her schedule before leaving for a month, I had too many scenarios running through my head up until the moment she told me the outcome of the test. She said they never give out the results (good or bad) over the phone. She scheduled a time on the first day in August when I could meet her at her office in San Francisco.

I thought I'd been holding it together when that horrible day arrived. It was an average morning. I washed my organic strawberries and blueberries and added them to my bowl as the foundation of my daily dose of antioxidants. I added four teaspoons of vanilla macaroon granola, half a Yoplait lemon yogurt and enjoyed the parfait along with a cup of jasmine green tea that offered additional antioxidants.

Years before, in her cancer research, Michelle had encouraged me to consume foods with higher levels of antioxidants: nature's way to help prevent the disease. I checked my e-mail and surfed the internet to distract my thoughts away from the day's meeting. I enjoyed the morning quiet before my children stirred.

A short while later, I looked up at the ceiling. I heard Sophie moving around up in her room. A muffled pounce, pounce, pounce echoed down into the kitchen as she jumped out of bed and ran to the hall bathroom.

A moment later, Mark entered the kitchen, readying to leave with our daughter. He was going to take her to her last swim lesson of the summer.

"Make sure she has some warmer clothes today since we're going into the city," I told him. "She can't wear a strappy summer dress."

"Yes, okay," he responded.

"What's the weather been like in the city lately? Cold?" I asked.

"Yeah, the fog has been making it chilly," he described typical summer weather in San Francisco that leaves unprepared tourists' lips blue.

"Hi, sweetie," I said to my little naked girl as she entered the kitchen looking for her bathing suit for the swim lesson.

"Hi, mommy," she said in a subdued tone, tired from staying up too late the night before.

"Do you have your clothes for later?" I asked.

"Yeah." She held up a pink skirt and a blue T-shirt.

"Sweetie, let's get a different shirt to wear with that." She began fussing and complaining.

"No, I just want to wear this, mommy. I don't want to change."

"Little girl, we're going to the museum this afternoon. Let's at least find a shirt that matches your skirt. Don't you want to look pretty?" I made the mistake of finishing with a question, thereby opening up the discussion to a debate with my child who negotiates every possible thing; she'll grow up to be a lawyer or politician, I'm sure. I grabbed her clothes before we walked up the stairs to her room.

When I was a little girl and my mom would drag us to museums in the city (I appreciate them much more now), she always had us wear stylish dresses, a fancy coat, Mary Jane patent-leather shoes, stockings and sometimes white gloves and a fashionable hat to match the outfit.

Afterward, we might attend afternoon tea at the grand garden court at the Palace Hotel, or go over to the Fairmont Hotel high up on Nob Hill where we would ride the glass elevator to the top of the hotel's tower. We would dine in the Crown Room looking out over beautiful San Francisco landscape. Sometimes, we'd go have a snack in the museum restaurant or stop in at Mama's restaurant in the basement at Macy's on Stockton Street for a juicy burger.

And if we happened to be walking around Union Square and dad was with us, he'd always buy corsages for all of his girls at a flower stand that had been there since the time my mom was a child. There was the one stand that always had violets, or my favorite, a gardenia. Oddly enough, Michelle's corsage always died quickly.

We'd walk through the shops. Mom would take us to Gump's where she and countless brides in San Francisco had registered for elegant wedding gifts. Just as my mom had done when she was engaged to be wed, we'd stroll through the aisles of tables exquisitely adorned for a formal dinner. She'd ask us what styles we preferred. She would take us into the jewelry room where my sisters and I would "ooh" and "aw" as we gazed at the lovely pearls and grandma's favorite, the jade. I would dream about someday registering for beautiful wedding gifts of my own: silver candelabras, crystal stemware and fine china.

"We're going to the museum?" Sophie got excited. It made sense to her that she needed a matching shirt. We went to her room to pick out a nicer outfit.

"Do you have your towel?" I asked her upon our return to the kitchen.

She fussed at me, "Yes, mommy. Right here."

"Okay. Let's put it in your bag." I reached for her clothes to put them into the bottom of the small sack.

"No, mommy. I don't do it like that. I put the towel in first."

"Sophie, that doesn't make any sense. You'll get your clothes wet trying to get your towel out of the bag. Here." I tried putting the clothes in first and she grabbed at them, yanking them out of my hands.

"But I always do it this way!" she got louder.

As my daughter yelled at me, all the morning's calmness fled my mind.

"Just do it, Sophie," I snapped back and crammed her clothes and towel into the canvas, pull-string bag. She stopped yelling at me and sat on a chair where she began crying quietly and whimpering in such an annoying fashion it was like nails on a chalkboard; she wouldn't cease her kvetching (kvetch: Yiddish for complain).

During her mini-tantrum, I returned to my chair in front of my computer and tried to push down the stress building inside me, but she wouldn't stop whining. The stress that had been building up over the past few months was about to culminate in this poorly chosen battle with my daughter.

I rose from my chair, walked over to her, and grabbed her chin to secure her gaze only inches away from my face. I growled through my words.

"Today is not the day to act this way, Sophie. You can't do this today. This lady I'm seeing today is going to give me one word that will change everything in my life and affect you and your brother. *One* word. That's all she's going to need to say to change everything. Do you understand?"

Of course she didn't understand. *She's seven and you're a bitch for treating her this way.* I was someone else; I was watching this scene play out, and I couldn't believe it was happening. I couldn't stop this train wreck.

I had to hold back from being more frightening than I already appeared, scarring her memory with one more neurotic mommy moment. Sophie's concerned expression made me pull away and sit down in a chair next to her. *Fix this. Fix this!* I calmed myself.

"Sweetie, come here." She sat on my lap and looked at me with a furrowed brow. "Mommy took a test in the beginning of the summer and I'm going to find out the answer today. It's got me a little stressed and scared. I'm sorry I yelled at you. But please, can you try to be a really good girl today?"

"Yes, mommy. Sorry, mommy."

I felt horrible having revealed this beastly side of myself to my baby girl.

The fight with Sophie left me anxious and crying. I wasn't mad at her, just worried for her future; what I was handing down to my children; the legacy of my father's mutated genes.

Mark traveled north to Santa Rosa with the kids. It was decided, he would bring them into San Francisco where they would meet up with me and my mom at Beth's office with enough time to hear the news before he had to leave for work.

By the time I drove away from our home, I knew it wouldn't take much to trigger tears. All morning, I'd managed not to think about how that day's results would affect my children. I continually told myself, this information was no big deal; I would just deal with it, but the argument with Sophie kept my children fresh on my mind.

Too many thoughts ran through my head during the drive south to my parent's home. I would stop there to get my mom. She wanted to be with me when I was handed the verdict.

I'd been driving southbound on the highway for nearly 20 minutes from our home in Sonoma County heading toward Marin when I looked around and realized I'd lost track of where I was. It took a moment to determine how far I'd already driven.

How will this affect Sophie? Will she have to have everything cut out of her like my sister, like me, if the mutation is inside my body? Will she be able to find love if she can't bear children, or if she has no breasts? Or will she keep them and live like a cancer time bomb?

And what about Jesse? What cancers will he be prone to? It's either prostate or colon cancer. I don't want to remember which. It turned out to be both. *Will he live a full, happy life?*

A mile or so before exiting the highway, I managed to get trapped behind a filthy truck hauling two porta-potties. The right one was painted beige with a rounded roof. The one to the left was painted brown on the front, green of the other sides and was topped with an A-framed roof.

I continued to be trapped behind this truck as I exited the highway and we traveled along the winding road.

"This seems apropos," I said to no one in the car. *Is this supposed to be ironic for the way my life will turn out after this meeting?* I further analyzed the porta-potty colors.

"And why paint them colors that remind you of shit and piss?" Eventually, the truck turned down another road.

As I continued along my route, I passed several women walking with their kids. Their children sat in strollers or walked alongside them. I thought about my own children.

In my heart, I knew the result of this genetic test.

"This is going to be a difficult year." I pulled around the corner and into my parent's driveway. I parked out of the way of my sister's car and was glad my mom was driving us into the city.

That thought alone should tell you how freaked out I was about these results. *I'll just close my eyes or look down, then I won't watch her poor driving abilities.* I entered the house to find my parents in the kitchen.

"Where's Michelle?" I asked after greeting mom and dad with kisses.

"Still in bed. Where else?" My mom's sarcasm pointed out my sister's haywire body clock. Generally, she can't get to sleep. She stays up most of the night and well into the early morning. When she finally manages to fall asleep, she sleeps in until late morning like a teenager.

"I'm back here," she called out from her darkened room; the guest room she took over several months prior when she returned home for cancer treatments and the various surgeries. She had wanted to return to Los Angeles to proceed with treatments and so on, but mom and I convinced her, she shouldn't go through the cancer on her own. Michelle dragged herself out of bed; her eyes were half-shut. Looking more like an old woman hunched over with a hangover, she walked to the bathroom down the hall.

"So, you sure you don't want me to come?" asked Michelle in a scratchy voice. I dreaded this moment I knew would be revisited following a similar offer during a phone conversation a few days prior.

While standing next to me near the hallway entrance, my mom whispered to me, "She just wants to help you, Joey."

"No!" Okay, too quick; a tad too loud. "No, no." Better; more nonchalant. "I'm sorry, Michelle. I know you want to be there for me but," I called out to her, *but I just can't deal with your hyperactivity today,* "right now, I just want my…my mommy." Everyone laughed.

"Mommy?" my mom said. "I'm tired of being mommy to everyone."

I thought about what lay before me this day and said I would understand if she didn't want to come along.

"I can handle it, mom. I can go myself if you don't want to." That's bullshit. I dreadfully wanted her there. "I know you've dealt with a lot of shit lately, so it's okay." I paused before lightheartedly adding a guilt-ridden, "That's okay," I sighed. "Don't worry about me." I brought up the back of my hand to meet my forehead and sighed.

Everyone fussed and laughed at my dramatic guilt moment.

"No, honey, I want to go with you," mom said. She looked around to make sure dad couldn't hear before whispering, "I really want to get out of the house and away from everyone."

"Oh, okay. Are you sure you don't mind driving? I don't think I should drive today."

"No. It will be better since I have the handicap plates and we can park anywhere."

That plan didn't work, anyway. Once we arrived at the medical center in San Francisco an hour later, we wouldn't be able to find any street parking. I would treat for the $20 parking fee in the lot across the street.

It is extortion, really, especially when you consider the people who use the garage mostly are cancer patients or their visitors at the hospital. If you are there for little more than an hour, the way they price it, you'll end up paying the 20 bucks.

I followed mom into her bedroom where she found her shoes and a jacket. We sat on the bed for a moment while she lifted her foot to rest on her knee. She worked her shoe onto her foot. She's one of those people who hold onto the sole of a shoe when they place it on their foot. That always bothered me. In my mind, I picture all the disgusting things people step in; it's on the bottom of their shoes, and then it's transferred to their hands. Yuck! I have to look away or down; anywhere so I don't think about the germs crawling around on her palms and fingers.

"How are you holding up, mom? Are we going to find you sitting in the bath tub again?" The last time Michelle had cancer and everyone thought she was going to die, one day, my mom reached her emotional limit. My dad's diabetes was impacting his health, and my (maternal) grandparent's health was beginning to fail. Mom couldn't take anymore and she was found sitting in the tub in her clothes; rocking and muttering and crying. That episode prompted a visit from her sister who flew out from Ohio to help with all the family's health crap and give mom a break for a week.

We've had too much shit in our family, and everyone needs a break.

Mom and I returned to the kitchen to find my sister sitting at the country pine table. She and I have similar taste, and I have the same table sitting in my house. It's funny. We both like our extra-long tables that extend to nine feet long when both leaves are installed because we envisioned large family meals; a gregarious bunch, everyone lounging, chatting and sharing stories. Ironically, our family has been shrinking.

"I think what you're doing is great, Joe," my sister was starting to wake up, but still held her head in her hands.

"I don't know," I shrugged.

"What do you mean?"

"I just…Why know if they can't do anything about it?"

"You don't know that," mom said.

"I'm just saying, I would want to know," Michelle said and looked at our mother. "I'd want to know," she repeated, then looked back at me. "If you know, you'll be prepared and you may not have to go through what I did."

"I know it's good for prevention, but what if they *do* find out I have this mutation? Then what? Then, I live my life waiting for it to happen? Waiting for cancer? I'd rather not know. I'd rather not live knowing I could get struck by cancer at any time," I told them.

"You think if the Jews in Poland knew what the Nazi's were doing—knew they were killing off all the Jews—they'd still say they didn't want to know?" my mother asked.

"Why must everything be linked to the Holocaust?" I asked.

"If they knew what was going to happen, don't you think they would have done something about it?" she continued.

"I thought they did have some information coming in. They didn't move on it," I said.

"Well…yes, but they didn't all know, and they waited too long because they didn't want to lose their things. Always remember; screw all the crap. Grab your kids, get out and screw the house and all the shit. If they had listened, they would have lived," she said. "Those Nazi bastards. You know, Hitler won."

"What do you mean?" I asked.

"The little prick won. I learned all the genetic stuff in that class Kaiser made me and dad take before we could find out if we had the gene. It's because he killed so many Jews. Now, the gene pool has thinned out and caused all sorts of issues in our genes. The bastard won!"

"See? Isn't it a good thing I married a Southern Methodist?" I asked.

"Yes!" my mom was excited. "We need his strong Scottish genes!"

"I knew there was a reason I fell in love with his stout, little legs," I commented.

"That's what you fell in love with?" my sister asked.

"Well, it was actually his…," my words were cut off by my

mother.

"I don't think I want to hear this."

"…Sense of humor," I finished.

"Oh," mom said, relieved.

"The secret to a successful marriage; keep each other laughing," I added, *as opposed to constant bickering and fights like you and dad…don't say that out loud. Don't say that out loud.*

"That and a good shtup," mom added with a hint of carnal lust.

"Mom! Is that all you think about?"

"Well, I can't help it. Your father's health stole that away," she whined. "I feel cheated. If only your father could have controlled what he ate, we wouldn't be in this mess. Believe it or not, your father and I were hot and heavy…."

"Mom, we don't need to hear this again," I said.

"Ooh, your dad and I—when we were younger—we were always screwing and…."

"Mom! Eew. Do we really need to hear this?" I covered my ears and made "la, la, la" sounds to avoid hearing about how horny they were as a younger couple.

"All right," she conceded.

"Mom, you need to get laid."

"Joey," she fussed. *Right. After hearing about your private sexual revolution, you're going to get upset by that?*

"We'd all be better off if you did," I muttered to my sister. She reaffirmed the sentiment by looking at me with raised eyebrow.

"At least your children will be better off with your husband's genes inside them," mom said.

Uhg. Back to that.

"Yeah. And at least you'll know if you have this thing in you," added my sister.

"I don't want to know this thing over which I have no control; this knowledge that is going to fuck up my kids' lives."

"You'd rather wait until it sneaks up on you and kills you?" Michelle fussed.

"No, I'd rather not have the damn thing at all and be able to live my life with my family."

"Well, *that's* the way to avoid dying," Michelle said in a sisterly snippy manner.

I knew I could never know all the range of emotions and turmoil my sister has faced through her breast cancer experiences, but neither can she climb into my head and understand why I didn't want to know the results.

Perhaps it's just being familiar with my pessimistic soul; I can base my fear of knowing this truth on my generally glass-half-empty outlook on the world.

Yes, I've had one sister who has already died, and that's when most people start echoing the well-established mantra to appreciate every day and live it as if it's your last. Fuck that. I was 12 when my best friend in the world was yanked out of my life. The horrible experience didn't turn me into a cheery person.

Yes, life is precious. Yes, life is short. And blah, blah, fucking blah...I know these things. I also know my kids are already growing up so quickly and may be required to face my legacy of mutated genes. And while I don't want to get cancer, I also don't want to live in fear of becoming its victim. Certainly, worrying about getting cancer can't be healthy. I know I've read somewhere that you can make yourself sick by continuously worrying about something. Isn't that just as damaging as avoiding it altogether?

"Let's just see what happens," said mom. "You may not have it and then you don't have to worry about it at all."

Just as I can run through a long succession of too many negative "what if" scenarios, my mom is equally efficient at producing a long list of what could go right.

Of course, she generally takes it a step beyond into the absolute impossibility of positivity after the logic train has left the building; I find her rosy interpretations rather annoying and frustrating. Either she has a positive attitude, or it's just one more way she finds to contradict my thoughts.

She's expert at finding the opposite argument to mine. Sometimes I trap her in her own skewed "logic," but otherwise, she spends most of her imaginary time on planet hyperbole.

We finally left the house.

During the drive into the city, mom and I fell easily into conversation with no need for the radio to fill in empty gaps. My sister always complains about this conversational relationship I have with our mother.

"I call, and you barely speak to me, but you talk to mom and you can't find a break to hang up even after an hour of talking," Michelle complains to me on a regular basis.

I know Michelle is lonely, not having many friends with whom to chat. Regrettably, once Michelle grabs hold of a conversation, she won't let go; she monopolizes any subject with absolute opinions that must be argued, on her part, to exhaustion.

The kids, Jesse especially, have become accustomed to flashing a certain look when auntie is lecturing on any subject matter; her favorite being the cost of living and the value of money.

"Say you get paid $1,500 a month. What would you do with this money?" During these conversations, Jesse tries to speak, but apparently this is a rhetorical question. "First, you have to pay your rent, let's say, $900, if you're lucky. Of course, in California, that will only get you a shitty, little studio apartment in a crappy section of town."

"Auntie said a bad word!" Sophie shouts.

"Oops, you're right. Auntie is bad," she admits before continuing. "Then, do you have a car?"

"Sure I do. I have a...," again Jesse attempts to answer by offering his current dream car. He's interrupted.

"You have to pay for insurance, gas, upkeep. And there's the cost of other things like phone bills, and medical insurance, and clothes, and food and...," the endless list continues until Sophie is lost in singing a song and Jesse looks bored out of his mind; and all because he made a typical child's comment to me about buying something for him because, "it only costs $10."

"I thought you like politics?" she'd ask me at another time when I would keep my answers brief, or say I didn't want to talk about anything political.

"Yes, I do." After all, I received my bachelor's in political science and worked in Congress on Capitol Hill, campaigns and the like. Only, she's never fully grasped the idea of a shared dialogue. Typically, she leaves little or no room for others to join in discourse when she pontificates on any subject.

But with mom, especially at times like these when we are alone and chatting about anything (including politics), it's easy to talk to her; we can joke around and diminish stress.

"I don't think I'm a good wife," mom said in the car. I burst out laughing.

"Can I quote you on that?" I responded.

"I don't care."

Out of my purse, I removed a small notebook and pen. *I don't think I'm a good wife,* I wrote down.

"Why do you think that?"

"Because all I want to do is get away from your father."

She told me about puddles of pee left on the floor when he misses the toilet. He leaves wet towels everywhere after showers. When he doesn't wear shoes to protect his abnormally, puffy feet (swollen due to heart issues), he bleeds on her white carpets. *Mom, I told you not to get white carpets.*

I tried not to pay attention to all the cars passing us on the highway. I managed to limit the number of times I had to remind my mother—who thinks cruise control is evil and, yes, too controlling—to push her foot down on the gas pedal. *Look down. Just keep looking down and play the game on your phone.* Regardless of the highway speed limit set at 65 mph, or 35 mph in town, mom drives one speed: 50 mph.

We continued chatting about nothing in particular and anything distracting until I asked, "It's good she wants to see me, right? She wants to offer some relief before she leaves on her big trip, right?"

"I don't know, Joey. Let's just wait and see."

Focusing our conversation on the elephant in the car triggered the first quiet moment since we closed the doors at her house.

"It could be good news. After all, you tested negative, so I have a fifty-fifty chance," I told her and tried to convince myself. I couldn't stop asking questions and listing various scenarios about why Beth wanted to see me before she left on her trip.

We got so lost in our conversation, I just barely made my appointment, leaving only a few minutes to spare.

During the many months leading up to this day, mom had become so accustomed to driving my sister or dad to their medical appointments at the VA or elsewhere, she instinctively drove toward 19th Avenue.

Lost in our conversation, mom didn't realize we were headed in the opposite direction until I commented about a childhood visit to the area. I glanced away from the game on my phone, looked down a side street and said, "Going this way always makes me want to get almond cookies from that place we went to when we were kids."

I briefly reminisced about going to one of many secret locals' spots for specific items like those scrumptious cookies. Suddenly, I felt famished. I thought my hunger could be a byproduct of my anxiety about heading into this meeting.

Unfortunately, after my innocent comment, my mom spouted,

"Oh shit! I can't believe I did this."

"What?"

"I'm so used to going this way. Damn it. We're going the wrong way. We're heading in the opposite direction of the hospital," she said.

"Do we have enough time to get there?" Prior to my comment, we were 20 minutes early, but now I feared we'd arrive late if we had to cross town through busy city streets. "Should I call them to let them know we'll be late?"

"No, I think we'll be okay," mom determined. She was right. We made the appointment on time after "Hal" directed us through San Francisco. That was the name she gave to the guy speaking in her car's navigation system, referring to the HAL computer in the movie *2001: A Space Odyssey*.

Leaving a few minutes to spare before my noon appointment, we arrived at my genetic counselor's reception desk. I signed in and ran to the bathroom.

"Do you want to fill out an anonymous survey?" my mom asked when I returned.

"What is it asking questions about?" I asked the receptionist. In so many words, she explained the results were meant to provide insight into patients' psyche prior to their finding out the results of their genetic test for cancer mutations.

"Sure, why not." I picked up the transparent, purple-tinted clipboard that secured the six-page survey and carried it over to a chair near the far wall. Mom followed and sat down next to me.

"What are they asking?" mom inquired.

"Oh, if I want to commit suicide and stuff."

"No. Really?" She didn't believe me.

"Yeah. Look." I showed her the survey before returning it to my lap and reading the questions to her. We laughed about some of the questions while I provided sarcastic responses.

Of course, my acerbic façade was my way of better dealing with the stressful meeting due to start a few moments later; the meeting that had the potential of changing my life forever.

Don't think about it. Just laugh.

Just as I turned over the stapled packet revealing the final page of questions, Beth entered the reception area and called my name.

"Oh, just two more questions."

"Go right ahead. We appreciate you doing this, so take your

time," Beth said.

"Circle all that apply," I read out loud to mom and continued, "In the past two weeks, have you experienced days when you felt 1) mentally well enough to accomplish many tasks, 2) upset and unable to accomplish more than a few tasks, 3) very upset and unable to accomplish more than a few tasks, 4) so depressed you were unable to accomplish anything." I circled all but number four.

The next question. "How often do you consider yourself: 1) a useful person, 2) not very worthy, 3) worth nothing."

Shit. They heard me. How many times have I told Mark I feel like a waste of skin?

"Okay. Done," I announced. Beth turned around after having been reading something up at the reception desk.

"Great. Let's go back to my office." Using her hand, she motioned the route.

Beth punched in a code on the security pad that opened a door leading to the back offices. She walked through the open door with me and mom following closely behind.

Hanging on the wall by the door was a hand-sanitizer dispenser that prompted a stress-induced Obsessive Compulsive Disorder (OCD) moment I hoped Beth wouldn't notice. In response to picking up that clipboard that so many others had touched, I quickly pressed my hand on the lower panel producing a squirt of sanitizer liquid to be released on my fingers curled under the dispenser.

I rubbed my hands together, distributing the gelatinous goo over my fingers trying to kill any germs transferred from the clipboard to my hands. I noticed, the slimy stuff had a different consistency and odor than my usual Purell and it took longer for the liquid to dry on my hands.

Having seen me take some of the sanitizer, mom didn't attempt to hide her motions when she, too, took some sanitizer from the hanging bottle. Her intentions were more overt than mine; for her, it was an effort to remain healthy and fend off any germs she may have come in contact with in the medical center. She had to prevent transporting potential illness home to my dad and sister whose immune systems were weak.

The depth of my intentions expanded beyond warding off potential illness; I had to rid myself of the transfer of, of...oh, shit, whatever had been left on that clipboard by the countless numbers of people who touched it before: germs, sadness, worry, tension, anger.

Psycho, I know.

"I'm so glad they have these all over this hospital. I think all hospitals should have those hanging everywhere to get rid of that coli stuff," mom said about the sanitizer.

Mom has her own language. "Biotics" are antibiotics, and "from-heetas" describes a meal at Chevy's: fajitas.

"E. Coli, mom," I corrected her.

"Right," she said.

We followed Beth through a maze of quiet hallways past offices hidden behind closed doors. As I followed her, my stomach began to feel sour.

It could be good news. You don't know. Maybe you got the healthier genes from your mother. You look like her, but you act like both of them; more logical like dad, though; perhaps, not so much right now, but most of the time, nonetheless. Yes, I know physical appearance has nothing to do with all this, but it's satisfying to think so, and mom doesn't have it! Maybe Michelle got the worst of it, and you'll be spared all the shit that goes along with her life! Michelle's always had the roughest road. Maybe she got all the shit genes, and I'll be spared. And why the hell not? I'm the fucking good child, damn it!

We walked through the door of Beth's office and sat down. The room was sparsely decorated; no real character or personal details; no photos of loved ones; no pictures of any kind. There only was a desk and office supplies, shelves, the basics. There were brochures that are supposed to offer help to those whose lives have just been crushed by destructive news.

Once all were seated—mom beside me and holding my hand—Beth didn't waste time to hit me with the news.

"Well," she started. Those were the last positive words I heard out of her mouth. "It turns out you *do* have the same gene as your dad. You don't have both, but the one you have is the same one your sister has."

I was BRCA1 positive.

That's it. I had it. The months of waiting for results had ended. I carried the fucker mutation; the little bastard. Mom and Beth's expressions showed concern. It felt as though I'd just received a death sentence.

"I do?" I don't know why, but I tried to remain calm. It was one of those moments when you're not sure how to react. No, that's the wrong description.

It's not on the same level, but it was like when I was a child and hearing the news that my sister was killed in a car accident. I thought, *what am I supposed to do? How am I supposed to react?* Our society is messed up if we don't know how to respond to intensely horrific news. Or, maybe it's just me.

Shit! Okay. I'm okay, so far. My momentary poise proved transient as my emotions began spinning out of control with the thought of my children and how this news would impact them.

I attempted to hold back my tears using my most contorted ugly-as-sin expression. I grit my teeth, pursed my lips and deeply furrowed my brow.

I couldn't speak, I couldn't scream. I couldn't do anything but look at Beth. Look at my mom. Look back at Beth.

Simultaneously, the terror-filled question pulsing through my mind was, *what about my kids? What have I done to my children?*

Too many things flashed through my mind, and they were all bad.

I saw visions of my sister's horrible breast cancer experience. What if my body is attacked by the disease and I die, leaving my kids to experience too much sorrow in their young lives?

I'm not as strong as my sister. I'd never survive what she went through. Worse still, my babies' childhoods would be ripped to shreds. What if my children carry this dreadful genetic mutation?

Oh, God...my daughter. What have I done to my daughter?

Will Sophie be able to have children? Will her ovaries be taken out and breasts cut off before she has a chance to meet someone and fall in love? Will she be able to find love if she is missing these parts that help define her as a woman and the mother of future generations? Will she choose not to have children because she won't want to pass on this mutation?

And my son. Will Jesse get prostate or other cancers? Will he carry this gene to his children and pass along this anguish of knowledge and experience?

I was overwhelmed. Only a couple words managed to claw their way out through all the horrible thoughts and escape my mouth.

"What about," I managed to say after what seemed forever.

"Yes, dear, what?" Beth asked quietly, leaning forward in her seat and displaying serious concern, compassion and patience. I could only complete my question in a whisper that fought its way through tears. My face grew hot; my head began to throb.

"What about...my kids?" I could barely say the words. "I only care about my kids. When can I have them tested to find out if...if they have it, too?"

"Well, we can't test them until they turn 18 and decide for themselves," Beth told me. Suddenly, the shoe was on the other foot.

"What? No! That's crap! First, you give me this shitty news. Then you tell me, I can't test my kids? Well, screw that! She made me do it," I exploded with frustration pointing at mom. "Why shouldn't I make *them* do it, too?"

Now I understand what my mother had been going through all those years whilst she's begged me to take the test. All those times I selfishly refused. I feel ashamed my compliance came only as the result of Michelle being diagnosed with her second breast cancer. I realized how impotent and helpless my mother felt.

I'm sorry, mom. Truly, I am. I'm so very sorry.

All the while, mom remained strong for me. She sat by my side, quite nicely filling her "mommy" role when I needed it most. She held my hand, looked warmly at my face with that exclusively maternal expression: she wanted to take away my pain, worrying, sorrow, anger, confusion.

"But what if they have the mutation and...must Sophie have a hysterectomy? She'll never...She'll never be able to...." These thoughts triggered a waterfall of tears.

For too many months since agreeing to have that genetic test, I had been suppressing tears and raging emotions.

Now, those months of repression were beating me into the nondescript rug in that monochromatic office. All the times I convinced myself there was nothing to worry about proved useless.

Beth and my mom spoke back and forth.

"Honey, there's such a small chance the kids have it because Mark isn't Jewish," my mom said. "I learned that in that genetics class Kaiser had me take when Dick and I were tested," she proudly told Beth who continued with mom's line of thinking.

"The possibility of them ever getting these cancers is at least 20 to 25 years away and we feel the decision to be tested should be left up to the children," explained Beth. "No one can tell them they have to do this."

"I will," I muttered, foolishly thinking I'll be able to influence them any more than my mother could impact my decision.

Beth told me my horrible odds of getting ovarian and breast cancers based on this mutation and my family history: my sister having it twice, and my dad's sister and mother both having had it.

Additionally, there were other members of dad's family who found out they carry the mutation, along with more cases of breast cancer. Our family had been targeted for painful deaths.

My chances of getting breast cancer were higher than 90 percent. Additionally, there was the likelihood of ovarian cancer. I was most assuredly doomed if I held onto the little cancer-plantation bitches in my body.

Most women have between a 1-in-60 to a 1-in-70 chance of getting ovarian cancer, I was told. Because of this genetic mutation, I was given a 1-in-3 likelihood of getting the silent killer. Generally, it knocks off women; by the time symptoms show up, the cancer is too far gone.

Beth and another nurse began explaining the series of appointments, tests, screenings and surgeries that would fill up my future. Add to that, I had to choose whether to cut out the parts of my body that are most vulnerable, or continue screening and hope for the best.

"You'll cut it all off. She'll cut it all off." My mother spoke to the two women as if she were telling the cashier at Nordstrom's she would purchase a pair of shoes her child had just tried on.

I couldn't escape thoughts about my children's futures.

"But what if they have it and they may get cancer?" I'd had my kids, so I didn't think I cared if they took out my ovaries and removed my tits. But what about my children? I was panicking.

"These cancers are not found in young children. Anyway, by the time they grow up, we'll likely have a better solution or a cure," Beth said.

Still, I found out later from a friend, that's the same thing they told her several years ago, and now her kids are in college. What's changed?

"Look. Right now, we need to concentrate on what you need to be doing and what your options are," I think I heard my mom and Beth consoling me.

"Okay. You're right. You're right, but this is really fucked up. I look like you," staring at my mom. "I was the good child, for Christ's sake!" I knew it was ridiculous to say these things, but I needed to say them.

Tissues. After drenching the small supply of tissues I had

crammed into my pockets for this meeting, I looked around Beth's office for more. *How can you hand out this type of information and not have any fucking tissues in your office? That's just cruel.*

After that, Beth began discussing the removal of my ovaries and fallopian tubes, thereby substantially reducing my likelihood of getting ovarian cancer. A prophylactic bilateral oophorectomy is preferred over the more traditional hysterectomy; the latter requires a significantly longer recovery. Of course, she added the caveat: there remains a small risk since they can't remove all those guileful, cancer-producing cells. She also spoke about having my breasts removed.

I think she asked what I wanted to do, but I couldn't focus on what they were saying; information had to be repeated.

Still, at the time, it seemed easy enough to tell them to go ahead and take my ovaries and tits.

"I've had my kids. I don't think Mark will care either way, so let's go ahead with it. Do what you need to keep me alive for my kids," I said, not realizing the full impact of what I was saying.

"This is the right thing to do, Joey. Just let them do this. You don't want to go through what your sister did, right?" my mom said to me.

"You're right, I know. No, I wouldn't survive what she went through," I said.

It was hard not to picture how weak Michelle became after the first breast cancer and how her body was ravaged by treatments and surgeries. She was always puking and could barely move off the couch. I had seen the dark rings around her eyes and the sadness in her soul.

I can't do that. I can't. I felt sick to my stomach, and then a new fear rushed through my body. *What if I already have cancer and it just isn't showing up yet? What if they don't get everything fast enough?* It would be my luck to schedule the surgery and the day prior find out that I have cancer, changing everything; changing the entire approach to my cancer-free future. My head ached from crying as these new fears pounded in my mind.

Our meeting dragged on beyond an hour during which another nurse came in to talk with me and then appointments had to be scheduled.

The best news I heard throughout the meeting was that if I chose to remove my breasts, there was a chance they could reconstruct them using my own fat.

"Cool," I said. I managed to calm down and focus on what they said for a moment. "I wouldn't mind that at all. Anyway, I've never been able to lose this," I said and used both hands to grab hold of my soft belly, baby-birthing fat. "I've had all this since Sophie was born. No, I wouldn't mind at all losing that."

Beth left the room to make appointments to have a diagnostic mammogram followed by a thorough clinical breast exam (those had painful written all over them).

Mark showed up with the kids at about 1 p.m. during the conversation about future necessary appointments. Unfortunately, the dates Beth found would require me to return to the city over the course of two days during the following week to meet with the breast surgeon, Dr. Laura Esserman, and the plastic surgeon, Dr. Robert Foster; both had been treating my sister throughout her cancer experience and they knew my family well.

Everything began moving so fast like I wasn't supposed to think about anything and simply jump head first into the "solution."

"Oh, but we're supposed to go camping next week. It's the only camping we've managed to fit into this entire summer." My spirits sank lower knowing we, or I, would miss going to one of our favorite camping spots; a place we return to every year with our children.

"I don't care about the damn camping," demanded mom. "This is more important than the fucking camping."

Mom's urgency didn't help with my constant "what if" scenarios filling my head.

"I know, it's just, the kids really have been looking forward to this all summer and...."

"Perhaps your husband can go up with the kids, and then you can join them later," Beth suggested. "Is it very far?"

"It's nearly to Mendocino," a couple hour drive from our home in Sonoma County, let alone adding another hour and a half drive from San Francisco.

"Oh, well, that's not too bad," Beth said not realizing the true length of the drive. After going to the campground on Monday, she suggested, "You could drive into the city on Tuesday and return on Wednesday. Then drive directly from the city so you can meet up again after the second appointment. Could you take Highway One?"

"No, that's even worse. It won't work." I thought of all the driving back and forth and only staying up north until Friday. We hadn't been able to book the reservation through the weekend because the campground was full.

"I suppose Mark could take the kids by himself, and I could stay home." Along with that idea, I noticed Mark wincing as a twinge of fear struck him.

Concurrently, I felt my spirits drop at the prospect of losing the opportunity to lounge around under a canopy provided by tall Redwoods. I would miss hiking with the kids, taking a picnic down to the river, or maybe some wine tasting at Husch and Navarro wineries to try out the current year's spectacular dessert wines. I would miss reading scary ghost stories around the campfire as the kids roasted marshmallows and made gooey s'mores.

Beth must have sensed the loss of hope. "You know what? Let me go talk to them again and see what we can work out." She left the room for a while.

Upon her return, she said she managed to fit me in for appointments during a single day. That way, I wouldn't have to stay in a hotel overnight to make the second appointment. The first was late morning, the second in the early afternoon, just after lunch.

"This is better," Beth said. "I don't think it's a good idea for you to be left home alone right now."

Perhaps she already read my answers in that survey and the question about if I have thoughts of ending it all. I don't think many people go through life without thinking about ending it now and again, but I've got kids whom I love dearly and certainly don't want to leave as the sole responsibility of my husband and family.

With the appointments scheduled, mom decided to take the kids across the street to a deli. She would feed them a late lunch while Mark and I spoke alone with Beth. My children wouldn't leave without first giving me warm hugs.

"I'm worried about you, mommy," said my extremely concerned son who tends to be like a mother hen.

"I know, but I don't want you to be," I told him. I held back tears, but I could tell he and Sophie noticed my puffy, red eyes. I tried not facing them too much in an effort to hide my sadness and fear.

Looking them in their eyes was too painful. Carried with the knowledge of this mutation was my father's heavy burden of guilt handed to me if I had passed along this killer mutation.

If Jesse and Sophie harbor this mutation, it may shorten their beautiful lives. I may become the cause of their bodies being mutilated by disease and treatments or the various prophylactic surgeries.

It's because of me their lives may be cut short. How can I do this to my children? They are extensions of my body and soul.

I burrowed my head against my son's chest as he stood in front of me. He wrapped his arms around my back and dropped his head to rest on my shoulder.

"Everything is going to be okay, sweetie," I tried my best to sound convincing. "Why don't you guys keep bubby company for a while and get her some lunch, okay? She's hungry. Are you hungry?"

They were. Asking that ordinary question; that was enough to distract little Sophie from the sadness expressed in my eyes and the agony ripping through my heart.

The three of them walked out. My mom spoke cheerfully to them as the door closed. Sophie began chatting away offering some story that would likely continue until they reached the deli.

They left, and Mark remained. He sat by my side and took over the hand-holding duty from my mom as Beth continued answering questions.

"I know this is a lot to deal with," Beth said.

"Actually, I feel ridiculous. Do most people react this way? Or am I just a total freak?" I directed to Beth.

"You know, with your family history, it's quite understandable that you should react this way." She didn't actually answer my question, but this was no time to start acting like a bulldog reporter.

I noticed Mark looking at his watch and realized how late it was. He had to get to work, and I wanted to go hug our children who were down the street joining their bubby for an afternoon nosh.

"I'm sorry. I have to get going," Mark said. It was okay. I knew he would only be able to spend a short while with me, and I preferred he take time off after my impending surgeries.

We said our goodbyes to Beth and walked out to the lobby where everything looked and felt different to me. I was exhausted and afraid. I felt the weight of stares as we left. I tried to hide my swollen, bloodshot eyes as we passed by patients waiting for their appointments in that cancer center.

I realized I was starving. Mark walked with me to the deli where we found mom chatting away with Sophie. When Jesse saw me, he came over to give me an enormous hug and held on tightly. My sight began blurring as tears welled up.

"It's okay, little bug. I'm okay. This is a good thing, kiddo. The doctors are going to make sure I stay okay," I spoke softly into his ear and his arms squeezed tighter around my back. "Say goodbye to daddy. He has to go to work."

My two boys exchanged a long hug and Mark reassured him everything was okay.

We walked over to mom and Sophie who sat by the window. Mom appeared captivated by Sophie's story.

My mom looked up at me with concern.

"Don't worry, Joey. Everything will be fine. You'll see. Just take care of this and everything will be fine," she told me.

Don't cry. Don't cry.

"I know. You're right," I responded. Her expression of concern remained. I avoided the subject. "Hey, I'm starving. You all got to eat, but I haven't had anything since breakfast."

Jesse jumped into action and offered to get a sandwich for me. Sophie said, "Look, mommy. Bubby got me some Cheetos and chocolate."

Mark left to go to work where he directs the evening news, and Sophie rushed me through my sandwich. She wanted to go do something fun in the city.

We decided to rush over to the Museum of Modern Art near the Moscone Center and fill the remainder of the day looking at paintings, sculptures and photographs.

The rest of the day slipped away, and always on my mind was what was yet to come.

After that difficult Friday, I was eager to be busy that weekend and distracted by packing and preparing for our camping trip starting Monday. I was glad to have time with my husband to talk about how this shitty mutation was going to impact our future.

Saturday evening after dinner, Mark and I were watching a TV show with the kids. As I sat in my chair, the sudden calm from the day's activities resulted in my mind racing with questions and too many "what if" scenarios.

I thought about the impending surgeries and the resulting pain.

I looked at my children and wondered how my BRCA status would impact their lives. Too many questions. Emotions brewed until I couldn't control my tears.

I got up from my chair and walked to the stairs. I covered my mouth and tried to conceal my rush of emotions as I climbed the steps and raced to our bedroom. I quietly closed the door and backed away, still trying to muffle the eruption of uncontrollable sobs.

A moment later, Mark came in and closed the door behind him. He walked over to me and took me into his arms. He held me as I cried. My body trembled.

"Tell me," is all he had to say.

"I hate this. I'm so scared. I hate knowing. I know I'm supposed to appreciate knowing so I can do something about this, but I can't stop thinking about it and what it's going to do to our lives. And I'm mad at my dad for passing on this fucking mutation to me. I know it's ridiculous to say that because he has no control over this, but I'm mad at him. It's stupid, but it's his fucking fault I'm in this position and Michelle has had cancer twice.

"I don't know what to do, and everyone wants me to rush into cutting everything off! But one minute I think, fuck it. I already have my kids and I have you. But I start thinking I'm crazy to take such drastic measures when I don't even have cancer. I don't have cancer! I don't have cancer, for fuck sake, therefore why am I doing this? What am I going to do? What's going to happen?" I continued crying.

Pounding aching took over my head; a stabbing sensation pierced through my forehead.

Mark held me and spoke calmly. "We're going to get through this. You're doing this to make sure you stay alive for our children, and we're going to get through this."

His words soothed my panicked mind. And on this day, our 16th wedding anniversary, his words managed to break through my fears and reveal another side of my husband.

I've always been one of those people who had troubles accepting that someone could love me. My sister Renee's sudden death when I was 12 left me realizing the frailty of life and not trusting people will stick around for the long haul; that lack of trust translates into not getting too close to anyone. Therefore, after 16 years of marriage, I still managed to question if my husband truly loved me. Why did he love me? In that moment, I experienced the depth of love he offered.

"You really *do* love me," I thought out loud. My surprise served to calm the dark thoughts controlling my future.

"Of course, I do," Mark responded softly.

"I don't think I ever realized how much until this moment." I felt grateful to have him as my husband and knew his strength would help carry us through the trying times that lay ahead.

CHAPTER 6:
ESCAPING REALITY

"Hi, mom? Can you hear me?" I spoke into my mobile phone.

I was sitting in our car's passenger seat waiting for Mark to finish busting up a solid lump of packed ice. We had just purchased the ice inside Lemon's Market in Philo, the small town a few miles away from Hendy Woods State Park where we were camping for a short week.

There was no phone reception at the campgrounds and it wasn't much better in town.

I tried to hear my mother's voice that competed with the racket of the bag of ice crashing against the rear bumper. Finally, Mark finished his task and poured the ice into the large cooler sitting in the back of our Ford Explorer.

Before having dialed, I'd been debating whether or not to make the call home to get an update on my dad's health. There was always something wrong with dad's health these days.

My sister had left a message saying dad was back in the hospital; this time, pneumonia.

Listening to Michelle's message that hot summer day, my stomach sank. I felt my body tense up as we drove through a forest of beautiful Redwood trees.

"Call your mom," Mark had told me on the drive into town.

"Do I have to?"

"Yes. You'll get more shit if you don't, so just make the call."

Before finally dialing mom's cell phone, I suddenly felt guilty for avoiding calling home to receive more distressing news, but only because lately, it had seemed most every time I called my parents, something was wrong. Someone's health was failing and they had to go to the hospital, my mom was mad at me for not doing more to help, or she was pissed at my dad because of his failing health.

I don't want you to have the idea that they don't love one another. Actually, my parents can be truly romantic and continue to love each other deeply after more than 50 years of marriage. Sure, they might bicker, but they also have fun together. But with dad's failing health, my parents transitioned into the stage of their marriage when one spouse takes care of the other; this would be frustrating and exhausting for most people.

Mom and dad joined the geriatric generation wherein the health care system forces this role upon people when (especially in California) it is too expensive to hire someone to help at $25 per hour, or move into an assisted living setting costing $7,000 per month. Eventually, these high costs would force my parents to move out of California where they could better afford their retirement and medical expenses.

Those few days at Hendy Woods had been relaxing and wonderful after having found out about that pernicious genetic mutation. It was always stewing in the back of my mind, but being away from home and reality helped clear my head.

I got to enjoy sitting in my "throne" at our favorite camping spot (no, I'm not going to say which one). Mark bought one of those outdoor lounge chairs for me so I can recline and look up at the trees and relax.

What a wonderful husband I have; he takes care of everything when we go camping. Ladies, if you want a man who takes care of you, find a Southern man. He's always busy doing something: making snacks or meals, mixing drinks, hanging out with the kids, making sure there's enough water in the popup tank, emptying the "juice box" from the toilet, and so on. It takes him a while to slow down and just sit, unwind.

When we weren't relaxing at the campgrounds, we would take drives out to Mendocino, always stopping at the Rock Stop where the owner remembers us from year to year.

Jesse picks out a fossil or some beautiful rock, and Sophie likes the little animals carved out of polished rocks.

Mendocino offered cool coastal relief from the scorching summer heat inland. We'd take a stroll along the weathered buildings housing shops that look out over the cliffs. We'd find a place to have dinner to give Mark a break from cooking over the barbecue.

We went to a restaurant—a fish-n-chips place—that has a balcony you can sit on and look out on the lawn and some historic building across the road. Just beyond the lawn, the land dropped off into rugged cliffs facing the ocean below.

After we ate our meal, Jesse and Sophie goofed around on the balcony, and I used my phone to take a photo of them. Jesse was standing behind Sophie, his fingers displaying bunny ears behind her head. Sophie was laughing and smiling. She has an innocence I've never seen on my son, or myself, for that matter.

That day, when I turned that picture into my screen shot on my phone, I didn't realize how much that photo would serve to cheer me up in the next couple years. The photo became my continued incentive and constant reminder of why I opted for surgeries.

But now, I had to call home and find out what was happening to my dad.

"Hello, Joey?"

"Mom, how's dad doing today?" I cringed, waiting for her response.

Either she would exhale a heavy sigh before listing her general difficulties, or she would be pissed I wasn't there to help. Worse still, her mood could swing in both directions. She would leave me confused, forcing me to choose my words very carefully.

My simple question triggered mom to react with tears and a dramatic urgency in her voice.

"Joey, dad has congestive heart failure," she couldn't finish the sentence without crying. I felt guilty after the thought ran through my head that I wished I hadn't made the call: the "responsible, loving daughter" call.

After all, we were away for these few days to escape reality at home and all the shit that lay before me upon my return. I felt lucky to get away after I nearly had to cancel my participation in our family holiday because of the meeting I'd had with Beth the Friday before. I felt lucky to have been given a reprieve from doctors' appointments and more grim news so I didn't have to toss my one chance at that summer's camping.

"Congestive heart failure? What does that mean for him, mom?" I was concerned.

"I knew he didn't look good. His ankles and legs were so swollen and...."

"Mom, what does this mean? What are they doing for him? Will he…will he be okay? What do the doctors say?"

"He could die from this, Joey," she cried louder now.

During the call, she was on the highway and driving to the hospital to see my father. I was concerned she wasn't focusing on her driving in busy Marin traffic. That same morning, she'd already had to deal with her elderly aunt's health.

Her aunt Toby, a widow with no children, had been protected by my mother's care for several years. Even though my grandparents had two daughters—mom and Donna—grandma made sure mom would always take care of her little sister.

Toby's mind had begun disappearing, impacted by Dementia, and no longer was it safe for her to live on her own. People who take advantage of the elderly were already beginning to prey on her.

That morning, Toby was taken from her apartment at an assisted living facility in San Rafael to the hospital. The facility had called mom saying Toby had fallen ill again, therefore mom met her at the hospital. Mom went in one direction while Michelle head over to the other hospital to check on dad until mom arrived.

"I'm getting so tired of all of this. I can't do this anymore." Pause. This could be her turning point where she chooses to go with the flow, or use me as a whipping post. "So how's your vacation going?" *Phew.* "I wish *I* could disappear on a vacation."

"I think you should." I really meant that. She needed a holiday from life's responsibilities.

"How are the kids? Are they having fun?" Speaking of the children minimally brightened her spirit enough to calm down and stop crying. My mother is the definition of a doting bubby.

"Yeah, they're fine. It's relaxing here. But, mom, what's next for dad?"

"Well, I don't understand why they don't have a heart doctor come in to see him if this had to do with his heart. Maybe Michelle's getting a heart doctor there now. I'm almost at the hospital." Toby's hospital was in a different part of the county from where Kaiser and dad were located.

"Come on, mom. If they haven't had a heart doctor there yet, you know what to do."

"What?"

"Just pull those balls out of your purse, shove them down your pants and get them to move their asses to get a doctor to check on him," I told her knowing her strong history of being aggressively proactive when it came to the health and wellbeing of her family members.

"Yeah, I know," she said.

Now for the dutiful daughter shit.

"Look, mom. We were returning home tomorrow, but do you want us to come home tonight?" I asked, knowing full well it would take us several hours to pack everything, close up the popup trailer and drive home.

Mom paused to think about this idea for a moment. Would my offer to sacrifice our holiday play in our favor? Or would this strategy backfire into the depths of "worst mistake in *Survivor* history" and force us to return early?

"I guess it's too late today." *Phew.* "What time are you planning on leaving tomorrow?"

"We have to pack everything and the popup and...."

"Well, don't take too long. I need you back here," impatience settled into my mother's voice.

"Don't worry. We have to be out of the campsite by noon anyway, and then it's a few hours to drive home."

"Okay. Don't worry about it tonight. Your aunt was nice." She spoke of her sister, Donna, who lives back East. "She offered to fly out."

"She just wants to get away from Eastern summer heat. So what's stopping her?"

"Naw. I told her not to. She was nearly struck by lightning when I was talking to her," mom spoke excitedly through a mood swing. "She was walking back to her car in the rain when she was talking to me, and after she screamed, I yelled 'Donna, what happened?' And when she got back on her phone, she said the lightning struck down right next to her."

"Right next to her? Maybe somebody is trying to tell her something," I responded with sarcasm.

"Well, it hit close by. She could've been killed."

"And you want to live back East? That's what you get with the weather back there," I told her.

Her focus returned to family drama.

"She said she remembered when grandpa got congestive heart failure. They pumped him full of medicines, and he pulled through it okay." Thank goodness; the sky isn't falling after all.

I had been tempted to call my sister before I called mom just to get a more realistic, drama-free, slightly more objective diagnosis of dad's situation. It's always difficult to distinguish reality from built-up fiction in my mother's tilted psyche.

"Well, see? He may not be as bad off as you think," I said.

Mom produced another cheery mood swing. "What are you guys doing today?"

"We're just hanging out at the campground, maybe a little hiking."

"All right." She didn't seem terribly interested. Again, she was distracted. "Just get back here when you can."

"Remember, we don't have cell reception in camp, so just leave a message on my phone. I'll listen when we leave tomorrow."

Before hanging up, I reminded her, she could call the ranger station if there was an emergency, or she could contact the local sheriff's department. If I don't repeatedly remind my mother of these types of things, it becomes my fault when she doesn't remember I gave her the information.

"What do I tell them? Where are you again?"

I repeated the details.

"I'm sorry I'm not there, mom. I love you."

"I know. I love you, too. Give the kids hugs for me and tell them I love them."

"Bubby loves you," I called back to the kids who were sitting patiently in the back seat of our car. The doors remained open to allow any possible breeze to cool the car as it sat in the sun.

Mark had since finished fiddling with the cooler and had climbed into the driver's seat, waiting for me to get off the phone. Mom and I hung up.

I realized my body had tensed up by the end of our conversation. My head ached and I felt my mood changing for the worse.

We went a few doors down to Libby's, the best Mexican restaurant in Sonoma and Mendocino counties. Libby makes delectable carnitas and al pastore; the best I've ever had. California has better Mexican restaurants than they do in Mexico and only a restaurant in Old Town San Diego rivals the food at Libby's. Yum!

The meal was great, but my stress level was tense.

During the drive back to the campgrounds, I felt annoyed by a song the kids began singing incessantly. The song's lyrics revealed its repetitive barrage of singing two words over and over until they ended the chorus with a hearty "yeeee haaaw!" And again.

If they didn't stop soon, brewing inside me was the snappy bitch resulting from family stress.

Don't children ever get bored of repeating things? I wanted them to be quiet. I had to talk with Mark about my dad's condition. After we had finished our conversation, the kids started singing again.

I realized I could get mad, or take another route and have fun with their childish behavior. I could enhance our camping trip memories instead of allowing a "psycho mommy" moment to put a damper on our fun.

"Where did you guys pick up this song?"

"On TV," they responded. *Of course.*

"You guys watch too much television," I said. They continued singing.

Another song with the same rhythm and complimentary tune popped into my head and I began singing in a high-pitched voice. It was *The Lion Sleeps Tonight.*

After singing the first couple lines, the kids stopped singing momentarily. "Keep singing!" I called out. They started up again, as did I.

The car windows were rolled down and we all started laughing; our sounds echoed off the forest walls lining the bumpy campground roadway. Slowly, Mark drove past the ranger's hut and then along the loop of campsites.

Our fellow campers interrupted their tasks to watch us pass by; to listen to the crazy folk singing with robust glee. Looking back at the kids, I could tell they felt relief; their faces relaxed. They were full of joy, comforted that mommy had chosen to sing over yet another spiraling-out-of-control angry funk after talking to bubby.

I was glad, too. We continued our singing and chatting as we took a hike through the campgrounds, down into the majestic Redwood tree grove and along the river.

We all simply wanted to enjoy our last full vacation day and the only camping trip of the summer before facing the reality of doctors' appointments, medical tests and surgeries.

CHAPTER 7:
THE NEWS IS OUT

When we returned from camping, we found the light on the answering machine blinking, announcing it was loaded with messages. The "cancer" calls had begun.

While we were gone camping, mom had told everyone in the family about my mutated genes, and now the relatives were calling. They were concerned; wanted to know how I was doing. Some were more demanding than others.

I called some of the cousins back. They all wanted to know what I was going to do. Clearly, mom had told the family, I would be cutting everything out as was *her* decision. After all, she gave birth to me meaning my body belongs to her, and not to me.

Some of my cousins understood my concerns with taking action versus leaving everything alone while continuing monitoring. They were kind and patient.

But as I expected, there was one cousin who would be more demanding in her choice for my future. She was the matriarch of our family who is married to the doctor of the family. It's not their real names, but we'll call them Golda and Noah. Golda was more intimidating than my mother.

"So, Joey. You're going to have a surgery to get rid of your ovaries and your breasts, right?" I didn't have a chance to respond. "So, when is that going to happen? Is it scheduled yet?"

"Well, I just found out a week ago and I've got some appointments set up already, but…."

"Where are you going?"

"UCSF."

"Oh, good. That's where your sister went, right?"

"Yes. I'm going to the same surgeons she did and...."

"So, when will they do the surgery? You *have* to do the surgery, Joey. We don't want to go through what your sister went through."

"I know, but...."

"But what? Don't put your mother through any more stress. With your sister and your father, she's got all the aggravation she can handle. Just get in there and take care of it, okay?"

"Yes, I know, but it's just all happening so fast and I know it's best for my kids, but...."

"But what?"

"I'm just freaked out by all this," I tried holding back tears, but failed. "I know I want to take care of it so I can be around for my kids when they grow up, but it's just so much to think about and I don't have to rush into it like Michelle did. I mean, I don't have cancer."

That was it. That was the source of my anger and guilt and frustration. How could I purposely mutilate my body? How could I risk dying on the table, knowing I don't have cancer and may never get it?

I'm not like one of those women sitting in the Breast Care Center waiting to see their doctor who will offer shitty news about their cancer progress. The women who will find out how fucked they are because the cancer wasn't detected early enough. Those are the women whose bodies will be thrashed by radiation treatments that likely will kill them after poisoning their system.

I wasn't one of those women who were told I only had a few months to live. I wasn't one of those women who knew some shitty little alien was eating away their body.

I wasn't my sister. I still had choices, but my family was insisting I only had one answer: cut everything out and hope you never get cancer because they missed some tiny, fucking, cancer-bitch cell.

"That's right, Joey. You don't have cancer and we want to keep it that way," Golda told me.

I listened to her words because my tears had silenced my voice.

"We just love you, Joey. You know that...," she spoke more soothingly.

"Mm, hm," I could only manage in response, shaking my head in affirmation. I dried my tears with my sleeve.

"And we only want what's best for you. So, you're going to go into the city with mom, right, and get this taken care of. Yes?"

I shook my head. "Mm, hm."

"Okay, sweetie. We love you. Now, you let us know what's happening and we'll do everything we can to help. We just love you guys, and your mom and dad, so very much and we just want what's best for you. Now, listen to your mother, okay?"

"I know. I love you, too."

We said our goodbyes and hung up.

Mark and the kids had been bringing camping gear in from the car. When they saw me crying, they stopped what they were doing.

"Mommy, are you okay?" asked Sophie. Jesse didn't say anything. He wrapped his arms around me and held on tightly. Mark rubbed my back, his face filled with concern.

"Yes, I'm sorry, you guys. Everything is okay. Everything will be okay." I pasted a smile on my face and tried to hide my bloodshot eyes. "Is everything out of the car?" I tried changing the subject.

"Almost," chimed Sophie. The kids returned outside to finish unpacking the car. Mark took me into his arms. I wiped my eyes on his shirt while I was sniffling loudly.

"Eew," he tried to lighten the mood, tugging the wet shirt away from his skin. His reaction made me smile for real this time.

"What's the big deal? That shirt is filthy from camping, anyway," I said, starting to laugh at his goofy expression.

"So, how many of *those* calls are on the machine?" Mark asked.

"Too many. Apparently, mom went ahead and alerted the media. And it gets better."

"What do you mean?" he asked.

"Listen to this." I pressed the play button on the answering machine.

"Hi Joelle, this is Rabbi...," we'll call him Rabbi Bernstein. He gave his phone number. "I was wondering if you might, uh, give me a call. Um, I'd like to hear from you and, uh, some information that's been going around." Oops. Quick recovery, "Nach, I shouldn't say it that way. I've been made aware of some situations regarding you, and I just thought maybe, you'd like to talk, um, so, I hope you'll call back. Again, the number is," he repeated the number, and then said cheerily, "Thanks, bye." Click.

I returned the rabbi's call.

"Hi, rabbi. This is Joelle Burnette."

"Hi, Joelle." A moment of uncomfortable silence.

"I'm sorry it took so long to get back to you. We were camp…."

"Oh, no, no. No problem. I just. I'd been hearing that you had a lot going on and…."

"Yeah."

"And that you have the cancer gene, and I just wanted you to know I'm available if you ever need to talk."

"I guess you heard from…," a friend I had confided in.

"Yes, she e-mailed me and said even though you are an atheist, perhaps I could help you."

"An atheist? Wow. I remember saying I have issues with God, but…."

"Don't we all," the rabbi broke in.

"But I don't recall considering myself an atheist." Indeed, never had I been labeled an atheist. And in that moment, I think I realized I couldn't entirely dismiss the idea of some larger force in our world. "Like I tell my mom; if I admit to having issues with God, then it must follow that I somehow believe in God, or something larger than us."

"Well, I know you have a lot on your plate and…."

"Yeah, my sister is on her second time with breast cancer and my dad is in the hospital and…."

"Your dad, yes."

"And I'm hoping he stays well because when Jesse has his Bar Mitzvah next year, he's the one person in the family who speaks Hebrew. Unlike the rest of us, he was raised orthodox back in New York City."

"Yes, well, there's a lot going on in your life. Jesse's Bar Mitzvah is coming up soon, and there will be planning and tutoring for that. When is he scheduled for?"

We spoke about Jesse's Bar Mitzvah for a few minutes, conveniently avoiding the more serious subjects.

"Well, if you need to talk or need any help, I'm here for you," the rabbi welcomed an end to our conversation.

"Thank you. I really appreciate it."

We said our goodbyes. After I hung up, I looked at the timer on the phone. It displayed just more than seven minutes.

As word spread, I heard from other relatives and I spoke with a few close friends in town about my decision to move forward with these surgeries that had my mind reeling in fear, anger and confusion.

Mostly, people thought what I was doing was brave. But one person questioned my decision.

My son and Harmony's daughter had been in the same classes since they were young. Over the years, Harmony and I had grown very close, and I considered her my best friend in town; the person I would call first when I needed help, or with whom to chat or hang out.

Also, she was the only person who questioned my choice to move ahead with chopping off my tits and removing my ovaries. And that was after I explained how the odds were against me.

"I just don't know why you would choose to take such extreme measures when there's nothing wrong with you. You don't have cancer and even with the high odds, that's no guarantee. You may never get cancer, so why do it?" she expressed in her honest, blunt style that usually I would appreciate.

Unfortunately, my mind was already whirling with general confusion and conflict. Her comments only served to make me more confused and feel crazy for taking these actions to secure my future.

It didn't matter to whom I was talking about my BRCA status and the surgeries; I couldn't help but to cry every time the subject was raised. I would even cry with the UCSF scheduling nurse when she gave me lists of all my appointments.

One time when she called, I couldn't stop crying. She said, "Maybe you should put off the surgery until you are more sure."

"No, no, I know I need to do this," I had replied through my blubbering.

Still, I questioned everything.

I questioned my choice to tell my doctors I would go ahead with the surgeries. I felt rushed in the decision; as though UCSF was treating me as if I were one of the hundreds of breast cancer patients who passed through their offices each week.

But I'm not like them, I would remind myself. I don't have cancer, and I may never get it. It seemed there was no urgency to my case. Therefore, why rush me into surgery as you would any cancer patient; the way you were forced to rush my sister to keep her from dying?

I'm not dying and I don't have cancer yet. I could get hit by a bus this same day and lose my life. Why am I doing this thing that will intentionally mutilate my body?

Even though I knew Harmony had a valid point and I tried explaining, again, how the odds were stacked against me, in the end, it all came down to one thing.

"But I'm doing this for my kids. I'm doing this so I can have a life with my children. I want to watch them grow into adults. I've seen what my sister went through with her cancers, and I don't want to go through that. I don't want my children to see that. I don't want to miss this opportunity to take control of this choice; one that cancer patients don't get. I want to be here for my children," I told her through tears.

But leave it to Harmony to find that one extra umph.

"What if you die on the table?"

Thanks for that. I paused.

"Then it won't be my problem anymore."

CHAPTER 8:
LOSING DAD?

One morning while dad was still in the hospital, I called my parent's home to see if mom had left to go be with him. My sister answered and told me mom was there already.

I said we would be driving down to see dad, but Michelle said she wasn't going that day. Understandably, she was tired. Of course as we found out later, her weak condition wasn't going to stop the sibling rivalry that had lasted all these years and into our 40s.

When we got to the hospital, mom was crying like dad was on his death bed (again). And repeating past complications, the doctors didn't know what medicines to give him that wouldn't negatively interact with his failing body. A blood clot in his neck required surgery; they needed to make his body stable enough to move him into the San Francisco Kaiser where the surgery could be performed.

As dad lay there, barely conscious, I stroked his hair back and away from his face. I quietly spoke to him.

"Hi, dad. The kids are here. How are you doing?"

His eyes were barely open. He didn't, or couldn't, respond. I kissed his cheek and looked up at my mom. She was worried and crying.

A short while later, to all of our surprise, in walked my sister. She took one look at our father and began asking questions of the nurse who made the mistake of checking on him at that moment while she was in the room. The nurse left, but Michelle came up with a task that must be carried out immediately.

She repeated this process, stomping in and out of the room in search of whatever she thought dad needed at that moment: a towel, more saline, a doctor, and so on. Her actions matched the general impatience she displays in most situations. Going behind a restaurant counter to pour her own drink or pick up her food from the kitchen are some of her classic moves when the waiters don't move fast enough for her.

In her distinctive "bull in a china shop" manner, when she returned to dad's room, she shoved her way past monitors and machines to go to his side and lean over so he could better see her face.

"Hi, dad. It's Michelle. How are you doing, dad?" she spoke in an unusually quiet tone to our father.

But it's what she did next that threw me over the edge.

Michelle gently clutched our father's hand; she picked it up and cupped his hand between her own. The simple motion would not have been unusual for most people, but this was my sister. This was someone who has never liked human touch from the time she was a baby. She didn't like to be held and her severe OCD prevented her from touching things, people.

But here she was, taking our father's hand.

"We love you dad. We're all here for you. Let your body do what it needs to," she continued.

The relationship my sister held with our father was marked by friction and fights, for the most part. Now, watching her holding his hand sent waves of emotion through me; suspicion, worry, doubt, sadness.

Based on Michelle's past, I couldn't discern if this small gesture of kindness was just an act; a way for my center-of-attention sister to attract a positive reaction out of my mother. *See, I'm here, too, mom...not just Joe*, I could hear running through her mind as she moved through the sadness in the room as if she was acting out a scene from a movie. Was she actually using our father's poor health to one-up me in what appeared a sibling-rivalry moment?

Generally, it wasn't her character to express this kind of human warmth. I felt slightly guilty for assuming this action was anything less than genuine. It must have taken a lot for her to do this, I considered, moving beyond her OCD reaction to touching most things.

Long before the days of people carrying around little bottles of hand sanitizer and while American parents still considered a little dirt in the diet as a healthy way to build up a child's immune system, ever since we were children, Michelle was the one who would wash her hands every few minutes to destroy anything that could be attracted to her hands by a simple touch; not just germs, but emotions and memories.

I was the child who always wanted hugs from my parents as opposed to my hyperactive, dyslexic sister who displayed autistic anti-social tendencies.

But now, in this moment when we didn't know if my father would live or die, my sister rose above her fear and dread of touch and took my father's hand in a moment of kindness and unanticipated warmth.

I was moved.

Her action left me terrified; perhaps this actually was the time for my father to die, I thought.

"I'll be back in a minute," I said and turned the corner outside his room and down the hall where I could better conceal my tears and fear of his death.

I had to find a private spot. Down the hall, I found an empty sitting room for patients' families. I hid inside. My mind wouldn't settle.

I reflected on my strong relationship with my father. I know he loves Michelle, but he and I have always had a stronger, more positive relationship. What if I didn't learn everything I could from him? I wondered if there was any advice I had missed. Do I know my father well enough for him to die now? What if there was something I missed? Perhaps a story that would reveal a new dimension of his character?

It was like walking into a college final exam thinking you might have missed something to study. What if I missed or I forget about that one thing he said that can make all the difference in my life, my future? What if there's more I need to know to pass along the memory of my father to my children and their children?

But then it struck me. I haven't missed my father's lessons. He's been a superb example for me. I've always looked up to him. I respect who he is as a man, a father, a husband. He's honorable and a good person. He loves us.

My husband came looking for me and mom followed behind. Michelle was off hunting down a nurse demanding something.

"What's wrong," mom asked.

I had trouble speaking through my tears. I waved my hand about as though I was communicating through the gesture, using the motion to prompt a flow of words from my uncooperative mouth.

"It's seeing him lying there like that. You and dad just mean so much to me and losing you would be...," my words ceased.

"What, honey," mom sat next to me with her hands caressing mine.

"Losing you or dad would leave my world so empty. I just don't know how I would be able to go on without you. With grandma and grandpa having died, I miss them so much, and I don't know how you do it all, mom. I don't know how you keep going without them in your life. And now with Michelle and dad sick...."

"Oh, Joey." She wrapped her arm around my shoulder and we cried.

"I'm sorry I'm crying. I didn't want you to worry."

"Joey, you know better than most, when it's your time to go, that's it," mom said, always referring to the useless death of my sister Renee within two weeks after her 19th birthday.

"I know, but...."

Using her mother's Jewish accent she said, "Sweetie, if your father is meant to live, then he'll live."

"I just hate seeing him like this." He was weak and grey, worn down by life's heavy boot. My children were too young to know him as I did. In his younger days, he was active, athletic and enjoyed life's treasures. His mind was ruled by sensible logic, and he was sought out for his intelligence and advice. He had a distinctly New York sarcastic wit. My children wouldn't know his true laugh and younger smile.

Sophie would grow up trying to avoid hugging the stinky, old guy: her grandpa who adores her existence. Jesse wouldn't get to hear stories about what it was like to grow up in the Bronx during the Depression, or how it felt to play basketball at Madison Square Garden and win the championship game for his high school, DeWitt Clinton.

And what if he doesn't get to watch his only grandson's Bar Mitzvah? He is so close to seeing that happen. Dad is extremely proud of his grandson for learning Hebrew and being such a mench. It was a significant milestone for my dad to see. Dad went through a lot of shit being a Jewish kid. It was important to my father that my children knew our ancient culture, qualities, values and pride.

Mom, Mark and I continued talking until we found something to laugh about and mom could finally, again, lovingly call her husband a shmuck.

The door opened and Michelle found us hiding in the little sitting room. She looked at us as though she had just discovered where everyone was concealed in a game of hide-and-seek.

"I was wondering where you all went. What's going on?" she asked. She was about to sit down, but we all stood up before returning to dad's room.

"Nothing," mom said. "Your sister's just upset about dad."

Michelle's body oozed hyperactivity as she looked at me with an expression that crosses the border from being inquisitive into desperation to be included.

We returned to dad's room to hang out for a while until the kids were getting bored and anxious to leave; their young metabolisms suddenly cried out for food. Additionally, Michelle's hyperactivity increased, and with it, she was annoying the nurses, the guy in the next bed, and anyone else who came near the room.

Understandably, after too many hospital stays—including her month stuck in the bone marrow transplant ward—Michelle doesn't do well in hospitals. The smells, sights, sounds. They all accumulate, leaving her nauseated when she walks through hospital doors. She becomes hyper, anxious, obnoxious, agitated, annoying.

But I get it. It's difficult for her. She said she's been told by her physicians this intense reaction is based on having post-traumatic stress disorder resulting from her first breast cancer experience.

We offered to bring back some food for mom, but she wasn't hungry and said she would get something later.

"I'll stay here with you, mom," Michelle offered.

"No, that's okay. Why don't you go with them? We should let dad rest," mom said. She and I noticed the guy in the next hospital bed was making noises specific to hints that we should gather up the family and get the hell out of the room; especially after Michelle said a nasty comment to him when he complained of Sophie speaking with some volume in her voice. The curtain separating the two men's beds didn't offer much privacy or peace.

"But I want to stay with you and dad," Michelle said. Mom gave me a semi-concealed "get your sister out of here" look.

"Why don't you walk us out, Michelle," I suggested.

"You guys go ahead," mom said. Jesse and I gave mom a hug, and kisses to dad before leaving.

"Where's *my* kiss?" Mark whined.

"Okay, I'll give you a kiss, too," mom said, and with that, Mark leaned in offering protruding, plump lips and a "mmmm." That always makes mom laugh and let out a boisterous "Eew!"

"Bye, bubby," Sophie said with zeal, offering a tight squeeze around her grandmother's waist. "Bye, papa," she called out to her grandpa. She wouldn't approach him to offer a kiss.

The next day, I called mom to find out about dad's condition.

"Hi, honey. Thanks for getting your sister out of there last night. She was driving everyone nuts," she told me.

"Okay, so she just left and didn't give any more hassles?"

"Yup. Whatever you said, it worked."

"She just wants to be there, mom. I told her, we understand why she has troubles being around hospitals, but she feels really guilty and just wants to know what's going on," I explained.

"She came into my room this morning and gave me a big hug and said, 'I love you mom.' She said she felt bad about last night. What is she feeling guilty about?"

"She said she didn't know about Renee's death until the doctor came out to tell her, she didn't know about her roommate from that group home jumping off the Golden Gate Bridge until months after the funeral, and she went off into the family room to watch M.A.S.H. when Daisy died that night." Daisy was our family dog: a massive, loving Saint Bernard who died in our garage the night before my parents were going to bring her to the vet to have her put out of her old-age misery.

"Daisy? Why is she bringing up Daisy?"

"She feels guilty she was watching TV and wasn't with her when she died."

"She wasn't there. We had gone out for dinner. When we got back, Daisy was dead."

"Oh, yeah. That's right," I said. "And now she feels like she's not going to be there for dad."

After that, mom said something after which I thought I would fall out of my chair.

"Your father and I decided years ago we have no guilt." *Please, qualify that one before the sky falls.* "No guilt about your sister's death. That's what kept us together all these years."

"Mom, Michelle says she feels left out of the loop because she didn't know Renee had died until she was at the hospital. I told her, at least she wasn't like me. I feel guilty because I was spending the night at a friend's house and having a good time when my sister was dying a few miles away. I feel guilty that I didn't feel something bad was going to happen to my most adored sister. I reminded Michelle, I didn't find out until the middle of the night when dad came to get me."

"Your sister doesn't remember. I think when it comes to death, she blocks things out," mom said.

I recalled, "As she did when she found out she had breast cancer that should have killed her the first time?" That day, all Michelle cared about was whether or not she was going to have scars on her breasts. Who gives a shit about the scars if you could be dying; that's what everyone tried telling her at the time.

"Yes. It's the same thing. She answered the phone call about your sister. She heard me scream, 'No, my daughter can't be dead!' She was in the car with us to go to the hospital and saw your father weeping. She just blocks it all out."

"I think she did that yesterday, mom, because she doesn't remember I told her on the phone that I was going down to the hospital. And then she just shows up. I think it was because I was going and she didn't want to be the shitty daughter that didn't help."

"Oy, and she just kept pestering the nurses," mom sighed.

"But she did just leave shortly after we left, right?"

"Yes. Thank you." Pause. "Well, at least now they're getting someone who can help. See? Your cousin was right. Dad needs a neurologist. Nobody ever listens to him, and nobody ever listens to me. I knew something was wrong. I should've been a doctor or something. I just know when people are sick. Like your ovaries, Joey. When are you meeting with them about taking them out?"

"Next month."

"In a month? That's too far away."

"Not in a month. In a few weeks," I sort of lied because I couldn't remember when I had that appointment set up with the gynecologic oncologist at UCSF.

"Oh, okay. It's just; I have a bad feeling about those ovaries, Joey. Not so much the breasts, but the ovaries need to be taken out."

"Yeah, I actually have the same feeling," I said. Mom and I share that strong connection in many parts of our lives. "Isn't that strange? I don't feel a threat with my boobs, but the ovaries have me concerned."

"Joey, you need to get those out soon. I just feel it. It's like the thing where you look for water."

"Dowsing?"

"I felt it in my body," she referred to the time she was given the opportunity to try her hand at using a divining rod. "Nobody listens to me, and I felt it then. I did that when I was visiting the Amish with your aunt that time. I felt very comfortable around the Amish."

"Okay, mom." Rein her back in.

"Well, at least they're getting a neurologist in there. Oh, shit!"

"What?" I asked.

"Christ! There's traffic backed up. I hate traffic."

"Okay, mom. Well, go drive and call me later with an update."

Eventually, dad's doctors decided not to do a surgery until they settled on a better plan. In the interim, dad was sent back into a rehabilitation center which caused more battles between mom and the health system.

The first place dad stayed was a horrible location in Petaluma. The Bay Area was experiencing high temperatures in the 80s and 90s and the heat accentuated the atrocious conditions in the rehab center that had no air conditioning. Several people were crammed into each room, and the high temperatures emphasized the nauseating odors of urine and feces.

In dad's small room, there were four men and one of the other guys had a urine bag that was leaking. The foul stench was enough to make you dizzy and want to vomit.

The food they served was atrocious. On dad's tray, they gave him Spam and canned peas. And for my diabetic father's dessert, these idiots provided canned fruit; the kind of fruit that is packed in sugary syrup.

"You can't eat this," mom complained.

Michelle took one look at the horrible food, picked up the tray and left the room to find a nurse. She slammed down the tray on a desk and soggy peas went flying.

"*You* eat this shit," Michelle demanded. The people in the rehab center were too sick to complain about the heat or the rubbish that was supposed to pass for food, she told the staff. This was one of the times I am glad to have a sister who is all action. The other poor souls in that place needed someone like her to stand up for them when they require it most.

Mom battled Kaiser to get dad out of there, and consequently, he only spent one day in the horrible setting. He was placed in another location in San Rafael near the Civic Center. He was alone in his room at this location, but the smell wasn't much better. Thankfully, the weather had cooled a bit, and this rehab center offered more air circulation; but still, no air conditioning to battle the hot days.

During a visit there, down the hall from dad's room there was a woman sitting in her wheelchair. She was alone in a room and repeatedly cried out for help. We found a caregiver, but they said, "Don't worry about her. She does that all the time."

Mom hated leaving dad in these places. After more fights with her health care provider, she found a caseworker who was helpful and kind. She managed to get dad into another rehab location. This one was much better; it offered superior care and conditions.

Dad stayed there for a couple weeks and eventually returned home to mom's care.

CHAPTER 9:
SOME LEVITY AND SUICIDE

"Watch out," I warned my husband who was sitting at the kitchen table near where my tea mug sat waiting for hot water from the kettle that had sounded a whistle after the water began boiling. He was looking at the computer and reading something.

In response to my warning, he said in a thick, slow Southern accent, "Is that hot?" Why is it, when he wants to act stupid, he thickens his North Carolina drawl, but he hates it when people assume Southerners aren't intelligent?

"Touch it and find out," I respond with sickly-sweet sarcasm. "Just think. When you're old and stupid with Alzheimer's, that's what you'll probably do." We laughed at that thought while I finished pouring the scolding water from the tea kettle. I returned the kettle to the stove, sat down, scooped up a spoonful of my Cheerios and raised it to eat. Mark spoke just after I placed the spoonful in my mouth.

"Of course, by then you'll take the kettle and go, "BAM!" right into my head!" Just when he said "BAM!" and swung his arm across his body, his action was such a surprise and funny, I uncontrollably spit out my cheerios and milk all over the laptop computer and Mark.

"Uuuuh!" he laughed and watched as I tried holding in the remainder of the cheerios in my mouth. I raced to the kitchen sink to spit it out.

"Oh, shit! I have to pee!" I was laughing so hard. He continued howling as I held my hand to my crotch like a young child running to the hall bathroom to empty my unusually-small bladder. No, really. Every nurse who has conducted an ultrasound on my belly comments on the small size.

"You could just see that happening in that evil little mind of yours, couldn't you?" he asked through his chuckles.

"I guess I had a *Dexter* moment going," I said when I returned. (Living under a rock, are you? *Dexter*: serial killer on Showtime. If the sight of real blood and bodily fluids didn't leave me so queasy, I'd probably make a spectacular psycho killer.) When I looked at the computer covered in a splatter of milk and chewed Cheerio bits, the result was a mixture of my unsavory snorting, laughing and crying.

"Oh, you told yourself a joke again, didn't you, and made yourself laugh, cry, laugh, cry. Oooh, there's a snort!" Mark made fun of me. Just then, Jesse walked into the kitchen.

"What's going on?" he asked with a smile.

"Mommy's making herself laugh again," Mark responded with a broad smile. "See what we have to look forward to, Jesse? Mommy's going to be a basket case when she gets her ovaries removed. And add menopause to that, and we're all in for a great ride."

I couldn't stop laughing and thought to myself how this is my favorite part of being married to this man. He always finds a way to make me laugh. These days, I manage to cry every time I talk about my BRCA surgery crap, ergo humor is a crucial ingredient to surviving this horrible process.

"Great," Jesse responds. "Eew, there's more," he says, pointing to the remaining milk stains on the computer screen.

Later that day, Mark called from work.

"I watched a man leap off the bridge on my way into work today." That's how my husband started off his conversation when calling from the television station where he works in San Francisco.

"Oh, my God. Did you...do anything?" I asked.

"Yeah. I kept driving. I can't stop on the bridge. It would create an accident. Anyway, it was on the left (east) side. It's always on the left side." That's the northbound side of the road. Mark was heading south into the city.

"Why always on the left?" In my inexperienced suicide mind, I thought, *gee, maybe they want to see the view of the city and bay instead of the ocean as they drop.* Even after living in the Bay Area most of my 40-plus years, I forgot, the west side was for bikes and the east side for pedestrians.

"What did you see?"

"A guy climbed up on the rail, he held onto the cables for a moment, some people rushed over to him, and then he jumped," he said matter-of-factly. "I watched him leap off just as I was driving by."

Neither of us could think what to say for a moment.

"Shit. Well, I hope you have a better day than that guy."

"Jesus, Joey."

"What? Obviously, he was having a really crappy day!" I worry about my husband and his extremely stressful job. I worry about the long drive he makes into the city every day; more than 100 miles of commuting. But I hope his days don't get so stressed and weighed down by too many pressures that he should end up like that guy and the countless others who dive off the Golden Gate Bridge every year.

"Did people stop their cars?" I asked.

"No."

"Did they at least slow down?"

"Yeah, mostly on the northbound side, but I was passing by just as gravity took him and any traffic stayed behind me." I couldn't believe I heard relief in my husband's voice; relief because this guy's shitty day didn't create any delays on his way to work. Who is the callous one now, right?

I was born and raised in the San Francisco Bay Area. I've driven across the Golden Gate Bridge for years (I've actually only walked half way across; that was back when I was in high school). Still, I've never seen anyone jump off the bridge. It's not that I want to. No, I don't want to. And yet, I wonder if my eyes would track their fall until the jumper's body smacked the water nearly 250 feet below the roadway.

I remember hearing the bodies of people slamming into glass after jumping from the Twin Towers of the World Trade Center in New York City after the 9-11 terrorist attacks. The sound was gruesomely graphic in that documentary filmed by a movie crew that happened to be following New York firefighters that day.

We watched the news throughout that dark day, and we were surprised the video actually showed people jumping to their deaths from those skyscrapers; they were trying to escape the raging fires that would engulf them if they remained. I felt sick to my stomach watching it. Yet, until their bodies were crushed and pulverized under the weight of falling concrete, I knew the people who remained in those burning offices would end up as "crispy critters."

Gruesome, I know, but it's a term my firefighter friends use.

Granted, the Golden Gate Bridge has a spectacular view of San Francisco and surrounding areas. Regardless, I've never thought that would be the way I'd want to die.

The surprisingly long fall would be just enough time to think you should not have jumped. And then, splat! But then what? You die frustrated so any of your ghost energy hangs around irritated, unhappy, unsatisfied and cold. Hey, it's windy on the bridge which is why locals don't usually walk across unless friends and relatives are visiting from out of town. Only the die-hard bicyclists cross the bridge over to the Marin Headlands or down into Sausalito and beyond.

I could just see myself sitting there, shivering, listening to other jumpers kvetch about their lives; bitching about their parents or something shitty an ex-lover did to them. Or these days, sniveling about their failed business or foreclosed homes. That *would* be hell.

You wouldn't be able to get away from them or their incessant complaining. You'd just sit there, down on the bulky cement platforms below the bridge, watching all the sailboats, happy wind surfers and cruise ships drifting by and think, *maybe this wasn't one of my best ideas.*

Then, of course, my mom would visit the location from which I flung myself to my death. She'd bitch and yell at me for shattering her life.

"Damn it, Joey. What the hell were you thinking? You're such a shmuck!" She'd call out over the side of the bridge as tourists would try to avoid eye contact. They would walk by quickly; anything to escape a potential conversation with one of those crazy Californians they'd been warned about by their neighbors back home in their safe Midwestern town and by Fox News.

That's if she wouldn't decide to join me by jumping after having gone through too much shit in her life (a lot of death and disease that reads like a Shakespearean tragedy).

Then, I'd never hear the end of it if her frustrated spirit followed me around for eternity on our cold, cement patch.

Still, at least my dad would have some peace and quiet having been left behind. Ah, but only after she yelled at him one last time and blamed him for their misfortune and for her just having hurt her hand after hitting the steel rail while she was expressing her anger at her shmuck of a daughter.

Sorry, I just leapt (excuse my poor taste) into my land of "what if." And before you think I'm a cold-hearted bitch and don't care about death, suicide, and so on, you need to know two things.

First, I've worked in politics and news where everyone pokes fun at intensely painful and sad moments. It's the only method of avoiding insanity (and jumping off the bridge) when you witness the horrible things that can happen; things that generally are edited from the news before stories are filtered to the public.

Consider the 1989 Loma Prieta earthquake that rocked San Francisco neighborhoods, bridges and overpasses just before the Oakland A's and the San Francisco Giants were to play in the third game of the World Series. I was working at KPIX-TV in San Francisco at the time. Even though we watched a driver smash down into a gaping hole in the Bay Bridge after part of the top deck fell down onto the deck below, I remember someone in the news room commenting on the driver's "floor it" approach as they attempted to fly over that missing stretch of roadway.

"Hey look, they think they're trying out for a part on *Dukes of Hazard*!" And yes, everyone laughed because it looked like a stunt driver's blooper when the weight of the car's engine thrust the vehicle downward into the hole as soon as the roadway disappeared.

So, I ask you, were we the brazen ones? Or should the guy who tried selling his video to every station in the city be ashamed? He was a tourist who happened to be crossing the bridge during the quake and was videotaping the scenery when he caught the accident on camera. Some stations turned him down—they don't pay for news—and others lowballed his offer.

After his excessive offer had been rejected by my bosses, I watched him walk through the newsroom looking pissed off.

Second, and more importantly, you've already read I have a sister who died. Therefore, I know what it is like to lose someone.

The closest connection I have with any bridge suicide is to know a woman who jumped. She had a shitty life; raped by her father, she was a runaway who took up drugs and sold her body to survive. She made her way into a group home and seemed to be changing her life around for the better. Still, it would appear the demons of her past took hold of her mind and spirit until she felt she had no other option than to jump off the bridge.

But bridge suicides like this young woman, or this man whom my husband witnessed jumping, would not become a story on the evening news.

"All the stations have an agreement they won't cover those stories," Mark told me. The stations won't make it a way for anyone to gain notoriety from their death. I'm surprised YouTube allows these videos. Do a search and you'll see; a little morbid curiosity.

CHAPTER 10:
EVERYONE IS DIFFERENT

The end of summer brought with it new schools for our children. Jesse was heading off into middle school. Sophie started at a new elementary school after her former campus was closed due to budget cuts. As we would find out later, we made the mistake of following the bulk of the students and teachers from the other school to her new school. As people predicted prior to the closing of the highly-regarded school, droves of parents removed their children from the district; the district was left with less money, translating into creating crowded classrooms and limited resources.

I had been very active at our children's former school and continued the same by going to PTA meetings and volunteering for various school events and activities as long as I was able. Doing those things had introduced me to some of my closest friends at their old school, and it made sense to do the same at their new campuses.

All the while, I had been going back and forth into the city. I would meet with surgeons, or have tests performed to see if my body's cancer factories has begun sneaking their evil poison inside me.

Mammograms, breast exams, blood tests, MRIs, oncological gynecology examinations, poking, prodding, discussions about reconstruction options, and appointment after appointment as everyone rushed me toward cutting off my tits and removing my ovaries and tubes.

Most of the time, waiting for appointments to meet with the surgeons meant waiting hours and hours to be seen. Sometimes it meant sitting in the exam rooms well into the evening and long after the front office had closed.

Thank heavens my invaluable friends came to the rescue to pick up Sophie from school or watch both my kids when my appointments dragged on unexpectedly and I was stuck in the city.

Mom wanted to be with me during most of the appointments. Sometimes she wanted to offer support and hang out with her daughter, but always, she wanted to hear what the surgeons were saying. And sometimes, these appointments became her escape from dad and Michelle.

She and I could chat for hours, and her presence helped those hours pass more quickly. It was comforting having her with me. Sure, there are times when we drive each other nuts, but most of the time, we have a friendship like none other; a friendship I treasure and will always hold dear to my heart.

Those days, chatting away and laughing, talking about politics or something silly, talking about the kids, making plans for the future or trips she wanted to take with dad; those days made the difference between running and hiding under a rock, and being able to face my future.

Mom was the perfect distraction to prevent my "what if" writer's mind from going mad. Instead of fearing my own future and the pain I was about to be handed, I would create stories about the women who waited for their appointments at Breast Care Center.

I'd see women walk in, quietly sign in and find a seat. They looked exhausted and sad; some, nearly beaten by cancer. Some women displayed the confidence they would survive their cancer. More revealed hints of terror.

And then there were those whose faces gave off no light. Their eyes were empty, their shoulders weighted by unfair and unfamiliar reality. Their bodies left to suffer unnatural medications meant to poison and kill. Those were the women whose clothes had become baggy because they had lost weight; they displayed neither energy nor hope; there was no point in buying more clothes to fit the thinner, unfamiliar version of themselves. Death clung to their back and waited for them to take their last breath.

These women would arrive with someone who was their support buddy who would sign them in while they found a few chairs to curl up on. Exhausted by the short walk into the cancer center, they would close their eyes and wait to be called by the nurse.

I stopped bringing books to read. Even though there wasn't anything to do while waiting for my turn to be taken through the doors and into the back offices, reading was useless. I found that I could read an entire page and have no idea what I had just read.

My mind was always racing with too many worries, concerns, plans, schedules, lists and lists and more fucking lists. Mom offered distraction while she thumbed through travel magazines and decided on another 50 places she'd like to visit. She'd make me look at photos on the pages.

"Joey, look at this. Isn't this beautiful? How would you like to go there? I wish your father's health was better so we could go to some of these places. See? Do these things while you can, because before you know it, your husband is old and can't go anywhere. Then, you'll be stuck like me." She didn't say this to be bitchy; she just wanted to have fun with the husband she loved.

Mostly, my mind was too distracted to concentrate on anything more than a game on my phone as we sat in waiting rooms or in the exam rooms. Hours, hours, hours of my life lost waiting for physicians. I kicked the shit out of Tetris, Snake and Bubble Burst!

They should have free video games in these types of waiting rooms. Bring in a Wii or something similar and give women a chance to race Mario Carts or shoot the crap out of some alien being to help defuse some of their cancer-related anger issues.

It was in these first few months after finding out I had the BRCA mutation that I went through a few cancelled surgery dates before the final date was set.

These cancellations weren't because of the surgeons' schedules. No. It was during these months when I went into a state of panic and confusion about decisions that would impact the remainder of my life. This was the time when I got information about my breast reconstruction options: implants, TRAM Flap, DIEP Flap, or no reconstruction at all and leave my chest flat and use prosthetic boobs.

Okay, I'm only going to say this once because I won't be able to remember what it stands for. TRAM is the acronym for Transverse Rectus Abdominis Myocutaneous (the last two words sound like characters out of a gladiator movie). Some simply refer to the "myocutaneous" as muscle. DIEP is the acronym for Deep Inferior Epigastric Perforator.

I'm not an expert, and I would advise anyone to speak with their surgeon or do research on the internet if they want the official definitions, but I'll tell you how it was explained to me.

If you're like me and have a double mastectomy, when you

have a TRAM, they slice open your stomach from side to side; one arc rounded upward above your belly button, and another arc rounded downward, with both arc ends meeting at your sides. Yes, you lose your belly button.

Then, after having removed all the meat of your breast tissue, leaving a thin layer of skin that will help form your new breast—skin that holds cells possessing the potential of becoming future cancer cells—they leave a 1- to 3-inch-diameter hole where your areolae and nipples had been. They will use those holes to attach that breast skin to the part of your body that used to be your abdomen. Oh, and they bore a hole under your chest to bring what had been your stomach up to your chest where it becomes your new breasts. (Confused yet?)

The reason why they bring the halved stomach sections up through your chest is so they can maintain blood flow from muscles that stretch out to accompany the skin/tissue chunks filling in the breasts. When they stitch everything back together, you have stomach-boobs and a tummy tuck. You also have to sit up all the time because of everything getting moved around; the stomach muscles require a lot of time to stretch up to your breasts. Everything feels extraordinarily tight after this surgery and will for many, many months.

This is a long, complicated procedure, but my surgeons said a TRAM is much more reliable than a DIEP Flap. In fact, they never offered a DIEP as a possibility. I had found out about the DIEP through a friend. I asked about it at my next appointment.

A DIEP, I was told, is less reliable because while they essentially use the same abdominal skin and subcutaneous tissue to form the breasts, they don't use the stomach muscles to maintain constant blood flow to the skin. Blood flow appears to be the key.

During a DIEP, they entirely detach the skin/fat chunks from the stomach region and use the severed mounds to recreate the breasts during the very long surgery. The surgeon (who requires additional specialized training) uses microscopic reconstructive surgical techniques to attach the blood vessels and return the blood flow to the new breasts. Unfortunately, if the blood flow fails, the re-attached flaps will essentially die.

Again, this is the information given to me. You should speak with your surgeon about these options for more official and medically-accurate information.

I'm told the benefit of a DIEP is that it is not as invasive and impactful to your stomach muscles. You can still do sit-ups, whereas with a TRAM, you no longer have the same muscle strength to do that exercise because the muscles that provide the strength to raise your torso from a laying position have been moved.

Unfortunately, the greater risk with the DIEP is that if the flap dies because the microsurgical technique didn't allow for proper blood flow, you'll end up with implants anyway. Then, you have to wonder why you went through all that suffering.

The odds of the skin dying appeared very low, yet it was enough of a chance to raise the questions asked by my surgeon. Would you want your surgery to be the one that doesn't work? Knowing you have a better chance with a TRAM, is the DIEP worth the higher risk of the skin dying and ending up with one or both breasts requiring implants?

That logic made sense and I tossed out the DIEP option, leaving the TRAM versus implants or no reconstruction.

I knew a week in the hospital while being pumped with pain killers after being sliced open from side to side translated into obvious high potential for suffering. Therefore, choosing this TRAM option over others may appear certifiably insane.

Still, after having seen what my sister experienced having breast implants after her mastectomies, I wasn't convinced choosing saline mounds was my best option. But that's just me, and here's why.

When my sister had cancer the first time, they took one breast. Her reconstruction options were limited to having no reconstruction (meaning a flat area where her breast used to be), or choosing an implant. Hmm. Such a choice, right? She chose the implant.

What you must understand is that when you get an implant, it doesn't just stay there forever. Over the period of a decade, her implant had to be replaced several times, generally because it popped or suffered other complications.

One time, while picking up my son and giving him a giant hug, for instance, she squeezed a little too tightly. Suddenly, she said an "uh oh" like most women might comment if their bra suddenly came unhooked. Her implant had popped. She had to go back under the knife.

Because of what Michelle had been through, I wasn't sold on implants, but the TRAM was frightening, as well. I frequently changed my mind about how to proceed and my surgery date kept changing because I couldn't choose a final reconstruction option.

I didn't think I minded losing my breasts. I'd already nursed both my children resulting in saggy mom boobs. Still, it was too much to consider. Every step translated into pain, and every time I had to discuss it, I ended up in tears.

Add to that, my sister made the mistake of showing me the gnarled, disfigured, scarred skin that remained after an infected expander had to be removed from her breast.

I remember when she was still in pain from the infection attacking her body, and she insisted on showing me what her chest looked like.

We had been at our parent's home discussing her health and the latest update on what the doctors were doing about her infected breast. She told me to follow her into the bathroom.

All of a sudden, without warning, she turned around, pulled up her shirt and showed me what was left of her breast. That summer day's brightness shined down on us through the skylight and made no effort to conceal any of the redness and ridges formed by the mangled skin that resembled raw ground chuck. I'm not one to shy away from a nude body, but this deformity sickened me and I had to look away.

"Oh, why did you show me that," I complained as I averted my eyes. The spectacle was burned into my memory and would become the focus of any fears of acquiring breast implants.

Time and again, my surgery was cancelled and everyone continued pressuring me to commit. Part of the problem was that I became an emotional basket case every time the surgery was discussed.

"This can't be a healthy way to approach a surgery," I told Dr. Esserman. "I read something that a patient is more likely to pull through a surgery and have a quicker recovery if they are mentally prepared for it. Clearly, I'm not in the right frame of mind." My doctor agreed and left my mother to protest.

And anyway, I needed some clear answers about the pain level and recovery time. I needed to hear something other than the standard line, "Everyone is different." This did nothing to calm my nerves. It made me feel like a piece of meat that had to be pushed through the surgical grinder with no consideration of my desire to understand how this surgery would impact my life.

I was given a DVD to watch that was supposed to help explain the reconstruction and recovery. I did try turning it on to watch at home, but quickly turned it off. It was too much to deal with. I couldn't watch it. *This is crazy. I'm crazy to be doing this surgery.* That DVD would sit by the TV for months until I could muster the courage to watch it.

Finally, a decision was made. Even though the surgeons said it would be easier to remove my ovaries and tubes at the same time they sliced me open for a TRAM, they would separate the surgeries; I would delay until my mind could better accept the colossal surgery I had to face.

For now, I would be scheduled to have my ovaries and tubes removed. The date was set. Thursday, October 16, 2008.

CHAPTER 11:
NO SENSE AND LESS SENSIBILITY

Since the beginning of the school year and prior to my first surgery, I had been trying to secure a job at Sophie's new school teaching the art enrichment program as I had done the year before. I had been in discussions with the principal, teachers and the PTA about how to bring to the program to the school.

In the process, other than telling a trusted friend who was a teacher, I was hopeful the school wouldn't find out about my impending surgeries. I didn't want that to impact the decision to hire me. Obviously, I feared they wouldn't choose me to teach the program if they knew I would require recovery time.

Once the first surgery was set to remove my ovaries and tubes and not include the double mastectomy, it came as a relief knowing the recovery time would be significantly shorter.

Before tackling my breast surgery, I would heal from the bilateral oophorectomy and my body would settle into its forced menopause.

Before the date was set, I had spoken with my mom about the art job. If I were trapped recovering from surgery, I was concerned I would lose the opportunity to teach.

"I don't give a shit about the job," my mom would express her frustration at my avoidance of reality. "Just have the damn surgery and get rid of it. Don't you understand how important this is? Dicky, tell her," she dragged my dad into the discussion.

"Come on, Joey. You know your mom is right. Just do it and get it done," dad said with calm insistence that didn't require mom's fervor.

"Yes, but I really want this job and if I go in for surgery, they're not going to want to hire me. I really loved teaching last year. I was good at it and the kids enjoyed the class. Even the teachers got together and figured out a way to pay me and...," I protested.

"And if you get cancer and die, the fucking job won't matter, will it," mom's trenchant comments cut to the quick. "What about your children? Do you want to leave them without a mother because you were worried about a job?"

"No, but...," she wouldn't let me finish.

"Who cares about all these other kids? You need to take care of yourself and get through this for your *own* children," she insisted.

She was right.

Getting the art job was important to me, but I also think it served as my escape from reality. I didn't want to think about the ghastly surgeries. I'd rather spend my days teaching art and having fun with the children. I'd rather watch their enthusiasm as they get to learn something new about the things that make life beautiful.

In the end, the job factor became irrelevant. The school district's budget was tightening because of California budget cuts. It was decided the PTA would freeze spending on anything extra in case they needed to direct the monies at necessary school supplies. These monies would become especially critical after the school's size had nearly doubled following the other school's closure that previous June.

No matter; I think I was a bit relieved considering what I faced in my future.

As the day for my surgery grew closer, once again, life became decidedly complicated.

In the beginning of October, Michelle went in for another surgery to have a new expander implanted into her breast. Yet again, within two weeks, another painful infection developed.

Also, dad was readmitted into Kaiser in Marin where, again, medication complications resulted in his being stuck in the hospital while they decided how to proceed. Moreover, doctors wanted to remove the blockage in dad's carotid artery to prevent another stroke. He was moved to the Kaiser in San Francisco where the surgery could be completed.

But my diabetes dad's health tends to be excessively susceptible to infection when he is hospitalized. His health began deteriorating to the point they were treating him for much more than the original issue for which he was admitted.

In preparation of my surgery, I was running back and forth into the city for tests, an ultrasound and various appointments with my surgeon, a gynecologic oncologist, and her support staff. Concurrently, mom was dealing with dad's health and Michelle was trying to secure help to get her growing pain under control.

The intensified agony she suffered resulted in her popping pain pills as if they were candy. Multiple times daily (sometimes hourly), she was taking 16 mg of Dilaudid, a derivative of Morphine. Michelle was showing signs of becoming addicted to the drug as her body built up resistance to its benefits. She was ingesting amounts that would render most people unconscious, but it had little impact on her. She proved hyper and agitated. And still, the intense suffering remained.

As I neared the day of my first surgery, there were concerns the laparoscopic procedure could turn into a bikini cut; the same used on women having a Caesarian section. Or in my case, repeating a slice made to my abdomen about 14 years prior when my gynecologist had to remove an extremely painful ovarian cyst the size of a softball. Because of its size, the cyst's removal required a longer slice instead of two small holes for a scope and tools used to remove a cyst. As a bonus, my doctor also found my appendix had shriveled up; remnants from my childhood and a visit to the emergency room when the doctors told my parents the discomfort I had been experiencing was not from an appendicitis. Guess they got that wrong.

There was a chance my surgeon's laparoscopic efforts to remove my ovaries and tubes might be hindered by scar tissue built up from my previous surgery. Now I had to worry about waking up with the severe pain resulting from a slice rather than a poke. I told my surgeon I'd rather repeat one of my difficult deliveries than feel that unforgiving pain again; especially if they would be slicing me open in a few months hence during breast reconstruction. The agony of childbirth is short-lived, but a slice produces constant, severe ache as the body heals.

Aside from those concerns, our family's doctors would be the first to deter people from jumping into surgery. Every time you go under the knife, there's always that chance that something will go wrong and you won't wake up.

Sometimes I wish my family wouldn't point out everything that can go wrong. I needed to focus on waking up and getting healthy so

I could continue being a mother to my children.

My children. That's what I thought about every time I needed reminding about why I was taking radical measures and joining a club of women known as previvors. We don't have cancer, thus we can't fight the disease. We previvors have a predisposition to cancer, but live in a grey area that can't be defined by certainty. Rather, we willingly choose to remove everything that likely will create the disease in our bodies as predetermined by generations of genetic material.

Until the day arrived when my surgeries removed these potential cancer incubators and I officially became a previvor, I would wake up every morning feeling like a cancer time bomb. Every day I would ask myself, is this the day I find out I have cancer and I regret having not moved quickly enough to cut out these cancer-brewing stations? And at the end of each day my mind would wonder if tomorrow would be the day I would get cancer.

It was exhausting. That's why I didn't want to know if I had this mutation.

Still, the day neared when my ovaries and tubes would be removed early on a Thursday morning in October.

In the days leading up to the surgery, I only wanted to spend as much time as possible with my children; just in case one of my many "what if" scenarios came true, and I didn't wake up.

But then my sister began causing problems for mom. I would be sucked into the next drama that Tuesday evening before my surgery.

"Will you please pick up your sister?" My mom was calling from the Kaiser in San Francisco, nearly an hour and a half away. I kicked myself for having picked up the phone that evening instead of ignoring the ringing and enjoying my time with my children. "She's doing her usual and driving everyone, and me, nuts." When Michelle gets revved up, she's like a wood pecker knocking on your head with a jackhammer.

"Mom, I'm not supposed to come near dad because he's having fevers, remember? They said, if he has an infection, they don't want me to going near him right before surgery," I reminded her about why I wasn't there already.

Even if I didn't catch something from dad, hospitals are notorious for spreading germs and infections. I shouldn't be going near the recovery wards within 36 hours of a surgery. Normally, it was mom who would be the first to tell others to stay away from a hospital when she knew they couldn't take the chance of getting sick; but because Michelle was involved, mom made allowances.

"You can stand out in the hall. Or call when you get here. She can meet you in front of the hospital. Joey, she's on so many drugs and in pain and shouldn't be driving. I'm staying here with dad, and I'm worried she'll get into an accident. Can you come get her? She's making me crazy, and I can't take much more of it."

This wasn't how I wanted to be spending my last evenings with my kids; picking up my sister because her anti-social behavior absent of filters or patience chased everyone away. Again, since her first breast cancer, this conduct was accentuated every time she walked through the doors of a hospital or doctor's office.

Wednesday was a school day and we didn't want to interrupt our children's routine; Mark and I thought if they remained busy in school and hung out with their friends, the distraction would help keep their mind off what was happening to mommy. Therefore, that left one more evening with my children. And as it turned out, my Wednesday evening would be spent running to the bathroom.

Before heading into this surgery, they have you evacuate your bowels. The way they do this is to have you drink this disgusting liquid that turns your evening into some repulsive episode of *South Park*. Oh, and when the nurse tells you, have a light dinner such as soup broth, take that advice to heart.

I made the mistake of eating a cheese burger because I had no self-control when my kids were eating theirs. I thought how bad could it be? Throughout the evening, I paid for my poor choice. It was horrible and painful to have liquid shit spraying out of your ass with the force of a power washer. The kids were already worried about my surgery the next morning, and this didn't help matters.

This added up to spending Tuesday evening sitting in the car during a long drive into the city. Granted, I was with my children, but that's not the same as being together in our home where I could better focus my attention on them. Instead, I had to take Michelle to the house in Marin before driving back to our home late at night just so the kids could go straight to bed. I would be left hoping they weren't thoroughly exhausted in school the next morning.

I called Mark and he said he could drive Michelle home that night after he finished directing the evening news. But because he wasn't going to be leaving the station until after midnight, Michelle wasn't satisfied with this idea. My husband had offered to pick her up at the hospital during his dinner break to bring her back to the station, but it was all too inconvenient for her.

"Michelle, all I want to do tonight is spend time with the kids before my surgery Thursday morning. Can't you let Mark drop you off?" I called and asked one more time. She would be stealing precious time when I could be holding my children while ensuring they knew everything was going to turn out for the best. When I was with them, I would control my fears and listen to their voices to fill my memory with happy sounds I could recall when I was put to sleep on the operating table. I didn't want to have my sister's manic speech running through my frustrated brain.

"But it's going to be so late before he can drive me home. Come on, Joe. Why is this such a fucking big deal?"

"Michelle, I'm not just driving down the street; it's going to be more than an hour to get there," I told her.

"That's okay. I can wait for you," she said. *Shit! This selfish bitch!* My mom took the phone from her.

"Joey, please. Do this for me. Hold on a second," she said. She walked into the hall and whispered into the phone. "Joey, I know this is an inconvenience, but please. She's driving me crazy. She's being rude to everyone; yelling at the doctors and nurses who are just trying to help your father. You know how she gets. I just need to get her out of here."

I knew well how Michelle behaved, especially in hospitals, and I couldn't turn down mom's request. "Okay, mom. I'll be there soon." We hung up.

"Come on, kids. We have to go," I called out to Jesse and Sophie who were playing in the living room.

"Where are we going?" asked Jesse.

"What's happening, mamma?" asked little Sophie.

"Bubby needs our help, and we have to go get auntie in the city."

"Now? But it's getting late." Even my 11-year-old son could figure out this wasn't the best idea.

I put my bra back on, changed out of my sweats and into regular clothes, and piled the kids into the car to drive into San Francisco.

"Mommy, why do you have to get auntie?" asked Sophie.

"Because your auntie always pulls this kind of crap and makes things inconvenient for everyone else, no matter the cost," I said, my anger and frustration growing. I was mad at my sister's selfish behavior. This was nothing new.

When I finally arrived in the city, we parked in the Kaiser parking lot and went inside the hospital. The evening left the hospital quiet. We found an elevator to the floor my dad's room was on and walked down the hall. Lights were off or dimmed in most rooms, and some patients were watching TV.

"Can I help you?" asked a nurse.

"I'm looking for my dad. Richard...?" There was no need to finish saying his name. I heard Michelle's voice as she rattled on about something. "Never mind. Thanks. I hear my sister."

We walked to dad's room and found him asleep. Mom sat flipping through a magazine and Michelle rattled on while playing a game on her phone. Mom responded, "Mm hm," never looking up from her magazine.

"Hi, bubby," Sophie said to get mom's attention.

"Ahh, there you are," mom looked relieved. Sophie offered a kiss and hug. Mom squeezed her tightly.

"Bubby, I can't breathe," Sophie said before mom released her granddaughter and repeated the warm greeting with her grandson.

"Hi, mom." I kissed her cheek, then asked, "How are you doing? How's dad doing?"

"Your dad keeps getting these fevers, so they can't operate on him yet. It would be too dangerous."

I looked at my frail father. He opened his eyes a bit. "Hi, dad." He didn't respond. My mom started offering a report about what was happening. I felt badly for my dad having people talk around him, but not including him in the conversation.

My sister began giving details she thought were necessary and complained about the staff until mom said, "Oh, enough, Michelle. Just give it a rest." Michelle rattled on.

Sensing my mother's frustration, I interrupted. "Mom, did you eat any dinner?" She had to think about it for a moment.

"Uh, I had a salad earlier down in the cafeteria. It was pretty good," she sounded surprised.

As soon as my children heard "cafeteria," they got excited that this could be an opportunity for a treat.

"Do you want me to go get something for you? Are you hungry? Want some coffee?" I asked.

"You know, why don't we let your father get some sleep and go get some coffee," she suggested.

"You guys want some ice cream?" my sister proposed to her niece and nephew.

Great. Not the best choice so late on a school night. Michelle saw my expression change.

"Oh, uh, if it's okay with your mom," she added the caveat that came too late.

"Please mommy, please," begged Sophie.

Thanks, sis.

Winding through halls to the elevator, Michelle walked ahead with Jesse and Sophie. My pace slowed when mom tugged on my arm; she wanted to speak without Michelle listening in. I put my arm around mom's shoulder.

"Oh, Joey. I'm so worried about your dad, and your sister is going nuts. She pops these pills, and they don't seem to do anything for her pain."

Maybe it was time to pull out the big guns and go safari on her ass! Get the elephant tranquilizer ready; this one's going to be a bitch to take down.

Michelle's hyperactive, nervous behavior was reaching its boiling point. So was everyone's patience. The stress and pain served as a catalyst for all her Tourette's idiosyncrasies to be revealed in rapid sequence: sniffling, huffs, snorts and various repetitive sounds.

"You should have heard her earlier. She fights with everyone and I'm left to deal with whatever's left. I know this was an inconvenience for you to do tonight, but I really appreciate it. She's driving me nuts, and I just can't take any more shit. I've got your dad in here. And I'm worried about your surgery," mom said as we strolled slowly.

We caught up with the gang waiting for us at the elevator and went down to the bottom floor to go to the cafeteria. The kids raced ahead and returned saying they were getting ready to close the food counters.

"Mom, what do you want? Why don't you sit down and I'll get you something," I told her. We found a table where she sat. She said she just wanted some coffee.

"Mommy, can we get a treat?" asked Sophie.

"Do you want an ice cream?" My sister did it again. At this point, I didn't care anymore. "Jesse, do you want an ice cream?"

Jesse doesn't have a sweet tooth like the rest of us and said he didn't want anything but something cold to drink.

I paid for his drink and mom's coffee before returning to the table where she and Jesse were sitting.

Michelle found some items to nosh on while Sophie finally made up her mind on an ice cream before bringing it over to the cashier where Michelle was paying for herself.

"Here, auntie," Sophie made the mistaken assumption that her aunt would pay for the unhealthy item she had suggested as a snack.

"Don't you have any money?" she asked her 7-year-old niece. "Part of growing up is carrying money with you and paying for yourself."

I couldn't believe my ears.

"Are you kidding me?" *You're so fucking cheap that* "you're not going to buy your 7-year-old niece an ice cream? One that you suggested she get?"

"I didn't know I was supposed to pay for it. I'm just trying to teach her a lesson about responsibility," she said. *Bullshit.* "Here," she added, slightly realizing her blunder. She dug through her purse looking for more money to pay the cashier.

Sophie was confused.

"Sophie, come here. Give this to the lady," I pulled $5 out of my wallet and gave it to her whilst Michelle continued to dig around in her tiny purse.

There I was, having just driven all the way into the city in order to chauffeur my sister back north to Marin and I said, "You can't pay for an ice cream for your niece without giving her a damn lecture?" I was getting so mad at her.

To begin with, she was carrying her wallet, which came as a surprise. Michelle had a reputation of offering to pay for a meal, or just for her own meal, and then conveniently forgetting her wallet at home. I'll get it next time, she'd say, or, I'll pay you when we get home. She rarely came through on those promises. Mark and I learned to expect this common oversight. She can be excessively generous in other ways with all of us, but she commonly forgets to carry cash. I can't say she does it on purpose; most of the time, simply she's forgetful.

"No, wait, here," said Michelle. She told Sophie to bring the money back to me.

Once they returned to the table, Jesse finished the homework he'd brought with him. I wanted Sophie to finish her ice cream so we could get the hell out of there. I'd had all I could take of my sister.

The increasingly irritated I became, the greater she acted as though nothing was wrong. She began spewing forth nervous small talk. I wanted nothing to do with her and chose to speak with my mom and let the kids talk to their aunt.

A while later, Sophie said she was getting tired.

"You guys better get home," mom said.

"Are you sure you're okay, mom," I asked.

"Yes, you get going." She knew the drive home was going to be a half hour longer because we had to drive out to the house to drop off my sister.

We walked to the elevators and parted ways as mom returned to dad's room and we marched out to the car. I started the engine and quickly turned on some music hoping I wouldn't have to talk to my sister. I was angry and needed to focus on my driving without getting into a fight with her. I drove west on Geary Boulevard toward Park Presidio Boulevard. From there, we head toward the Golden Gate Bridge and Highway 101 leading north to Marin County.

People who drive in a city like San Francisco tend to drive a bit aggressively, always on the defensive; more so than driving outside the bustling city. On occasion when returning home after one of my medical appointments, even mom appeared to think she was Steve McQueen acting out a scene from the 1968 movie *Bullitt*. Yes, there's nothing like watching a 70-something grandmother's minivan catching air in Pacific Heights on Divisadero Street while heading over the steep hills down toward Lombard Street. I didn't mind the views of the bay, but I generally found myself bracing my arms while hanging onto the dashboard and hoping my mother wouldn't kill us both. All the while, mom would be laughing, calling out, "Weee!" and asking, "Isn't this fun?" And she thinks I'm a terrible driver?

That evening, I wasn't driving in that dangerous manner, nor did the route I chose have steep hills. But later, when I looked back on how I drove that night, I do feel guilty for not applying a gentler disposition considering the pain my sister had been experiencing. Michelle was always in pain since the first cancer, but I didn't realize how agonizing her pain had become. (I'm genuinely sorry, sis.)

I was angry at her and didn't care about hitting bumps in the road. Nor did I take care to ease into a full stop at red lights or maneuver gently through traffic. Haven't you ever been infuriated by your sibling enough that you acted stupidly and full of spite? This was one of those times I've grown to regret. My driving wasn't enough to disturb the kids or put anyone in danger. Still, I wasn't adding extra care to make this inconvenient, stressful evening easy on my pain-in-the-ass sister.

I love my sister, but I don't always like being around her.

The quieter I became, the more Michelle tried to talk to me. I didn't want to fight with her and knew there was nothing I could say to make her understand the world doesn't revolve around her; other people have crap in their lives, too.

She pressed and pressed until finally, I made the mistake of saying, "Okay. You want to know why I'm so mad?"

We drove in the narrow lanes across the Golden Gate Bridge; the local landmark is always congested with heavy traffic. That probably wasn't the safest location to kick off this discussion, but I began anyway.

I said I understood she had too many burdens because of the cancer; more than I would ever be able to manage. Regardless, her problems didn't give her free license to add shit to the lives of everyone around her. Her actions and behavior have consequences; I thought she was being selfish this night because she's not the only one with worries, concerns, stress. I said she could have been dropped off by Mark who was already in the city. I told her, her timing sucked and how I just wanted to spend time with my children because I was worried about my surgery in less than two days.

She rattled away in an aggressive, nasty, condescending manner, and her voice became louder and louder. What did I have to worry about? I didn't have cancer, and this was, in her mind, just a quick, nothing surgery. She spoke in jealous terms, angry because I had Mark and she had no one. Again, what did I have to worry about?

She didn't want to hear a response; she only wanted to vent and yell and bicker and bitch. The louder and faster her speech became, the more I realized this fight wouldn't end well.

Jesse began calling out, "Auntie, stop fighting." With his words, I worried how this battle was frightening my children.

At these times when Michelle exhibits this manic behavior, I'm forced to call upon strategies that require I remain calm and speak soothingly until she settles into a rational dialogue. It's useless to match her yelling because she only grows louder and more frenzied. On this occasion, this soothing strategy proved ineffectual.

"Stop," I said. She kept going. "Okay, just stop. It's enough." She wouldn't stop, and I tried to remain cool-headed while focusing on driving on this busy highway.

By the time we neared the top of the grade and passed through the Waldo Tunnel that greets drivers with a rainbow painted over the top, Jesse and Sophie were crying; they were begging for an end to the fight.

"Please, just stop. You're scaring the kids. Michelle, stop! Just stop!" She wouldn't cease her rapid-fire rant about how shitty and selfish I was. "Stop, please stop," I begged. The government doesn't need to torture someone with water-boarding or round-the-clock rock music blaring; let Michelle get going, and she can make anyone crazy.

Any remaining patience fled my mind. I made the mistake of adding some volume to my voice. I continued to beseech her to stop. She only responded with louder ranting as she dispensed a constant flow of berating remarks while I drove in the highway's fast lane; I continued on the grade up from the tunnel and over the summit. As we began heading down the hill toward Sausalito, it was pure chaos in the car when my phone rang.

I answered the call and heard my husband's voice. Michelle demanded to know who it was. Even under the best circumstances, she didn't like people talking on the phone around her if she couldn't hear the conversation. Regardless of the caller or subject matter, she would insist the call be placed on speaker allowing her to hear what was said.

She had increasingly grown paranoid of people talking about her. My mom and I would explain it was none of her business to listen to a private conversation, but she would make issue of it every time the phone rang. Furthermore, if you didn't let her listen in, she'd insist on knowing everything that was said by the caller.

"Who is it," she yelled at me.

"It's Mark. Can you shut up for a minute so I can talk to my husband for Christ sake?"

Hearing it was Mark, Michelle yelled, "No! You're not going to talk to him and tell him shit about me! You're not going to make me look bad," she added and lunged for the phone I held to my ear.

As she lunged, she bumped into my side causing the car to swerve, nearly running into the center cement barrier as we rounded a narrow curve.

"STOP IT!" I yelled. "Are you trying to kill us?" I told Mark I'd call him later. The kids were sobbing in the back seat. Jesse held his hands to his ears and kept yelling to stop the fight.

Michelle continued yelling and ranting until I couldn't take anymore. I finally lost it and shrieked, "STOP!" I did this as forcefully as I could to get her to shut up. My outburst resulted in everyone momentarily growing quiet and my throat feeling sore. The kids continued sobbing.

At that moment, I just wanted her out of my car and out of my life. How many times was she going to act this way with me? I didn't want this crazy woman around my children. I wanted to get her out of my car.

I picked up the phone.

"Who are you calling?" She stopped ranting, but she was still acting suspicious and paranoid.

"I'm calling you a cab. I want you out of my fucking car" *you crazy bitch.* There was no point in yelling or speaking anymore. There was no reasoning with my lunatic sister and I just wanted to get her away from my family. I'd had enough of her psychotic, irrational behavior for which she rarely takes responsibility. I was tired of making excuses for her actions; I was tired of listening to my mother making excuses for her unreasonable conduct based on her shitty childhood, her dyslexia, her complicated adult life, or any other label she claimed had control over Michelle's emotions, mind, life, future.

In mom's mind, it seemed it was never Michelle's fault for anything that occurred. Repeatedly, I've tried explaining to mom that just because someone has issues, that doesn't eliminate the hurt they cause. But when mom considers Michelle's participation in conflicts, generally the blame falls on others; on anyone but my sister. Simultaneously, if you tried to offer details about an incident, mom simply would discredit reality with any number of excuses: Oh, that didn't happen. You're making it up. You're overreacting. You're too sensitive.

When we were children, Michelle had a rough time in school. She had troubles with her teachers who had no idea how to handle a dyslexic, hyperactive child. She got into many fights with the other children and often left school bearing bruises and other battle wounds. Many days upon returning home, her aggression and frustration from her lousy experiences were transferred to me. Well, fuck her if she thinks I'm going to allow her to be a deranged lunatic around my children. (My mom is mad at me for calling my sister deranged, but come on, mom. I've heard you call your own sister crazy on occasion; we siblings have our moments.)

I called information for a cab company. They connected me to a number, but no one answered that night.

"But I don't have enough money for a cab," she said.

"That's not my problem," I answered as we passed through San Rafael heading north to Novato.

I tried calling information again, but my luck didn't improve. By this time, we were nearing Novato. I wanted to dump her anywhere along the way to get her away from my children, but I knew mom would be upset (even though on occasion, she's been known to kick Michelle out of her own car).

I stopped talking to her.

She turned to the kids who now looked at her with fear in their eyes. She reached back to Jesse to pat his knee. I looked in the rear-view mirror and saw him flinch away from her touch.

She began realizing what she had done.

"Oh, shit. I'm sorry you guys. I didn't mean to scare you. Auntie loves you. I guess I fucked up. I didn't mean to scare you." In the faces of my children, she saw a small reflection of her actions. She began expressing regret, but it was too late; the damage had been done.

Sophie was still young enough that she might forget this fight after a while and still see her auntie as a fun playmate. Jesse was another story.

It would take a few years before he'd want to spend any time with her or confide in her, as he did prior to the big battle; their relationship would never be the same. For a long time, he was afraid to go near her and didn't want to go to my parent's home to sleep over if she was there. Before this incident, Michelle had been like an "Auntie Mame" to Jesse. After that, whenever he saw her, his innocent affection was transformed into dread and mistrust.

Before he would again offer warmth and affection to his aunt, it would take frequent conversations with him reminding how she genuinely loves him; she would do anything and everything to help him. I explained how auntie has some mind issues that make her act the way she does and treat people with little respect. I knew she would die for my children; I just didn't want her to kill everyone in the process.

My parent's home was near the end of a quiet cul-de-sac pushed back in Novato. As we neared their street, suddenly Michelle insisted I wait a moment while she went inside to get a birthday present she'd been making for me. My birthday wasn't for a couple of weeks.

"Michelle, I don't want anything from you," I spoke calmly. "I just want to get my kids home."

"I'll just be a minute," she said. "I've been working on this for a while, and I just want you to have it. Take a look at it and tell me if you still think I'm selfish. It's your birthday gift."

"I don't give a shit what it is. I don't want *anything* from you. I just want to go home," I repeated quietly, looking straight ahead. We were a few blocks from our destination and she began hunting for her house key.

We drove around the corner and I made the mistake of pulling half-way into the driveway. She jumped out and ran into the house as I backed out before circling the end of the cul-de-sac.

"Mommy, here she comes. Hurry," Jesse called out as though we were being chased by zombies.

Just as I was about to race away, Michelle ran in front of my car. I slammed on the brakes and we stopped. In one hand, she was holding a package rolled in newspaper. She used her free hand to strike the front of my car.

"Open your window," she yelled at me.

"Is she nuts?" I said to myself. I shook my head, no.

"Open the window," she called out again. "I want you to have this." I tried backing up, but there was no place to go. "I won't get out of the way until you take this."

I just wanted to get out of there. I opened the window just wide enough for the package to fit. I nearly threw it out the window, but I was afraid she would get angry again and do something to hurt us or smash my window.

"If I'm so selfish, why would I make this for you?" she yelled as I hit the gas.

I tossed the package onto the passenger seat where she had been sitting. I sped away from the house, leaving her in the street.

She was still yelling something.

I began driving home, but before we got back on the highway, I pulled into a nearby strip mall where I got the kids out of the car and gave them tight hugs and spoke to them for a few minutes. I wanted to make sure they were okay. They both cried, and Jesse said he hated his auntie.

"No, I don't want you to hate her. Auntie has a lot of problems, but I know she loves you. She may not always show it the right way, but I know she loves you," I told him. Regardless, he was still frightened of her.

We got back on the road, and we were all exhausted by the time we got home. I got the kids to bed before calling Mark to let him know what had happened. He said he was worried about us, and he was mad at my sister.

"So what did she give you?" he asked.

"I don't know. I haven't looked at it yet. I just don't give a shit."

He told me to see what it was. I removed the newsprint.

"Oh, wow," I said and started crying.

"What? What is it?"

"It's one of those 'Day of the Dead' statues I like. She painted it in the surrealistic style of a Rene Magritte," I described the vibrant colors and the gold trim. It was a ceramic skeleton woman wearing a full-length dress. The long skirt displayed a blue-sky scene with some clouds. Red and green apples were raining down to the bed of purple-flowering iris plants circling the bottom edge of the skirt. Michelle had used oil paints to blend and transition the light blue sky into darker night with polka-dot stars on the woman's blouse. She was beautiful.

Mark and I talked on. "You know I nearly threw it out the window at her? It would have been smashed to pieces. But what do I do with this? I feel sick looking at it. She's such an idiot."

I knew, every time I would look at this woman, I would remember that horrible fight. Likewise, the way she gave it to me—the timing of it after realizing she may have unreservedly screwed up and gone too far—it's like a husband giving his wife beautiful flowers or jewelry or something to show how much he loves her right after beating the crap out of her.

"Doesn't she get that?" I asked.

"No, and she never will. Your sister is psycho," said Mark.

"Damn. Why did she have to give that to me after a huge fight?" I truly felt sickened by the remarkable gift.

After our conversation had ended, I fulfilled the promise to my mom to call her once everyone was at home. I was going to keep it from her that we'd had our big fight, but she heard residue of frustration in my voice and sensed something had happened on the way home. She badgered me to reveal what had occurred. I didn't give her too many details other than we had a fight and Michelle frightened the kids with her behavior.

I told how she wouldn't let me leave without the "gift."

"Oh, Joey, isn't it beautiful? She's been working on that for months. She found that statue when we took her to Mexico on that trip. She knows you like those, so she wanted to make it special for you," mom explained. "You should tell her that you like it." *Fuck. Do I have to?*

"It's really beautiful, mom, but I wish she had waited to give it to me another time when we hadn't been fighting."

Next, I called Michelle. I told her the gift was stunning and how I had nearly thrown it out the window. I also told her how it felt to receive it under those circumstances. I tried setting it out on display, I said, but it made me ill to look at it because of how it came into my possession. The experience had tainted its beauty.

"So what are you going to do with it?" she asked.

There was nothing I could do other than pack it away in a shoe box. It would remain stored in my closet until I could look at the damn thing without feeling ill.

"Well, when will you display it?" She pressed for a precise amount of time that would pass.

"I don't know, Michelle. As long as it takes for me not to feel sick to my stomach when I look at it." She was frustrating me again. I couldn't believe she wasn't grasping why I couldn't leave it in view. She was more concerned about her piece getting attention and compliments. Her selfish concern disregarded any distress over what had happened and how that battle would now, thereafter be tied to that gift.

For several months after, every time we spoke, she would ask if I had displayed the statue. No. Why not? You know why; because it reminds me of that horrible night. How long will it take for you to put it out? When I stop thinking about the fight and simply want to look at it for its beauty, I'll display the piece. How long will that be?

She wouldn't make the connection. She couldn't understand how every time I looked at the dark, star-filled sky of the statue's blouse, I remembered that night filled with her verbal abuse and the way she terrified my children. She avoided the truth and tried to brush it off as if it meant nothing. It was the same every time. I had to ask her a few times to stop asking me. It took about a year for me to display the statue.

She wanted to know how the kids were. I told how she wasn't their favorite person.

"Shit, did I really fuck it up with them?" she asked.

"Sophie may forget, but Jesse doesn't want to be anywhere near you; at least for a while."

"Aw, crap," she responded.

"Michelle, what did you think was going to happen?" It was useless to try explaining, but I did. "You were acting like a crazy person, and all you did was scream at their mother most of the drive home, and nearly run us off the road in the process."

"Well, you said shit, too," she insisted.

"Yes, I did, because I thought you were being selfish, but...."

"It's because I'm in so much pain, Joe, and...."

"Yes, I know you are in pain, and I'm sorry that you are, but it doesn't give you the right to shit on everyone around you. I'll get over this, but think about what this did to the kids. You were screaming while they were begging you to stop. I was trying to get you to stop, but you kept going. And now the kids, and Mark...."

"What about Mark? Oh, shit, does he hate me now?" Reflecting my parent's affection for my husband, Michelle adores her brother-in-law and wants him to like her.

"What do you expect, Michelle? He's not going to jump to your rescue when your actions make things difficult for us or our children." I think she was more concerned about how Mark felt about her than how I did.

"This really wasn't how I wanted to spend this night with my kids, Michelle," I spoke with exhaustion in my voice. Since we were children, it always seemed everything had to be concentrated around my sister because of all her issues, her problems; it appeared little had changed. I knew it never will. I don't blame her for having started her life with learning disabilities and hyperactivity. But shit, even mentally-disabled children can be coached to have better social skills than my sister displays on too many occasions. (Yes, mom, that's one of my angry lines.)

Mom was worried about Michelle, dad and now, me, as I faced significant surgeries, but that didn't stop my sister from being a thorn in everyone's side at the hospital. Yes, she does deserve to have a better life free of pain and cancer, but she doesn't have the right to pull everyone down with her because of her actions.

I was facing this surgery in very little time and worried about the pain, recovery and simply being rendered unconscious. I feared the possibility that something could go seriously wrong; I'd leave behind my two beautiful children. Michelle couldn't grasp the depth of why I was so concerned. I hate to say it, but it's because she doesn't have children of her own. She doesn't know how that connection ties you to your babies; your children are part of you, and when they hurt, you hurt, and so on.

She's always said she can relate to animals better than people, and she'll say she loves her pets as much as I love my children. She has exhausted this comparison. One day, I finally told her, you adore your pets and say they are like your children. Regardless, you can't leave children locked up in an apartment for a week with a little extra food while you go on a trip.

I knew Michelle was worried about her own recovery, but she seemed to miss the point that everyone has crap in their life. Regardless, she expects people to jump when she needs something.

I managed to get off the phone before another battle began.

CHAPTER 12:
THE DOC FORGOT TO MENTION...

The day arrived when the surgeon would remove my ovaries and fallopian tubes. And after all the angst leading up to that early morning surgery, the scar tissue from my previous ovarian cyst surgery didn't impact the removal of my insides.

The same day I had the surgery, I was able to go home that afternoon and begin the healing process. With the pain medication, I didn't feel so bad; just some cramping. I spent the remainder of the evening in bed resting and sleeping.

Around dinner time, Mark took the kids with him to go get some food to bring back to our nest. I continued to sleep until I was awakened by an intensely sharp pain stabbing my shoulder. Yes, not in my abdomen, but my shoulder.

I began shifting my body, but that made it worse. Afraid to move, I called out for Mark. I didn't know what was happening. I couldn't understand why my shoulder was being attacked by a concentrated piercing sensation when it was my abdomen that should have been hurting.

I lay there in the dark screaming for Mark and crying from the intense pain that felt as though someone had sunk a knife in my shoulder.

A short while later, Mark came running into our room, he turned on the light and found me in tears.

He called the doctor's office, but the answering service would have to contact her.

Mark sat with me. He held the phone waiting for the doctor's call. The kids came into the room to find out what was happening. They looked concerned.

"Is mommy okay?" Jesse asked, "Why is she crying?"

Mark assured them mommy would be okay and sent them downstairs to eat their dinner.

Finally, the doctor's office called back.

Oh, that's pretty typical of a procedure like this, Mark was told. It was just some gas caught in my body. It sends a message through the nerves and impacts the shoulder. It would go away after a while.

Why the fuck didn't they tell me that before I had the surgery? I would have preferred to have been prepared to deal with this pain instead of being hit with a surprise attack.

When they conduct this laparoscopic procedure, they pump your abdomen with carbon dioxide (CO_2) gas to provide the surgeon a better view of your insides. Unfortunately, depending on their method, residual gas can impact your diaphragm and somehow affects the nerves that go up to your shoulder. The pain, I learned later, generally starts several hours after the surgery and dissipates as the gas works its way out of your body.

Mark was told to give me an over-the-counter medicine such as aspirin or Aleve, and to use a heating pad on my shoulder.

Eventually, the pain went away and the recovery began. I was told to take it easy for a couple of weeks and then I should be fine.

Almost immediately, my still youngish body was forced into all the symptoms common of surgically-induced menopause. I must admit, I welcomed the end of my menstrual cycle. Unfortunately, hot flashes, sleep disturbances and riding an emotional roller coaster were the most notable changes triggered by menopause. Later, there would be weight gain and other little things like my once-strong fingernails thinning out and revealing ridges.

Because of my high risk of cancer, I wasn't a candidate for hormone therapy. Therefore, my au natural menopausal journey was marked by frequent hot flashes; especially at night as soon as I would lie down.

It's an odd feeling, having a hot flash. It starts in your head as you feel your brain boil and your face get hot and red. The wave of heat travels down through your chest and you want to begin grabbing at your clothing because you just want to rip it away from your skin that quickly becomes covered in sweat. Often, when a doozy of a hot flash is about to strike, I'll suddenly feel sick to my stomach, and that queasy feeling washes over my body prior to the wave of heat.

When it happens in public, people look at you like you're

having a heart attack. They ask if you are okay. My hands would begin to tremble as I'd rip through my purse hunting for a fan I started carrying. I would whip it out to flutter and build up a gust of wind cooling my face and chest.

"Sorry. Hot flash," I don't know why, but I would apologize and feel as if I had to explain when I noticed peopled staring. It always happened at the worst times.

I kept fans in different parts of my house. Mom started buying pretty fans for me as gifts. I had one in the kitchen, another in the living room, one by the bed, and eventually, one in bed behind the pillow so I could grab it quickly in the dark.

Night was the worst time. The hot flashes would steal my sleep and comfort. The sweat was enough to bleach the color from my sheets. With the aid of hair scrunchies, I would wear my long, thick hair in a stack on the top of my head to keep the natural blanket off my neck that would leak like a sieve during a hot flash and soak my pillow with sweat. I could no longer wear a night shirt; I would awaken while tearing it off my body to escape the suffocating heat. Henceforth, I began sleeping topless.

We have a ceiling fan over the bed, and even though it was winter, I would keep the window open and the fan on high. All night, my body temperature seesawed from hot to cold, cold to hot. Our down comforter would blanket me when I felt chilled. But when I'd feel a wave of heat washing over my body, I would violently fling the comforter onto Mark in my desperation to cool down.

It wasn't long before this nightly battle with the sheets, the wind from the fan and the room's cool temperature impacted Mark's sleep, as well. My menopause chased my husband from my bed and into the spare room where he could get some much-needed rest.

On the emotional front, I felt as though I was becoming a manic depressive with euphoric highs and dismal lows. Laugh, cry, laugh, cry; it's exhausting and confusing. I was warned, my abrupt loss of estrogen would result in these intensified symptoms of menopause. That knowledge didn't make it any easier to deal with the symptoms.

And even though I knew I didn't want any more children, I now had to come to terms with this permanent termination of my fertility. It was odd being in this situation where the choice to have babies was sliced away, forever. I suppose it's like anything else; once you know you can't have it, suddenly you want it more.

I had to keep telling myself, what's the difference, you don't want more children. Your husband doesn't want more children.

In the months leading up to the surgery, and for several months thereafter, I found I became a bit melancholy when I would see women with their babies, or if I passed by a shop selling baby clothes. And then there were the comments mom would say without thinking.

"Oh, isn't that adorable," she'd comment while looking at baby clothes. "Maybe you'll get pregnant, and we can buy that."

Her casual comments were especially difficult to hear after my ovaries were removed and left me a little sad, but I knew she meant no harm. She had to get used to the idea I could no longer get pregnant.

While I convalesced at home after my surgery, mom was still running into San Francisco. She would stay with my dad, and help my sister who was trying to get her doctors to address the growing pain she was experiencing in the area of her breast expander.

Over the course of several days, Michelle had been trying to get help to ease this pain. And actually, I feel like a total shit as I admit the following: the night of our big fight was at the end of a very long day for Michelle as she tried to secure that help and was sent home. Clearly, her frustration accentuated her actions during our battle.

That day, mom had driven Michelle into the city and left her at Mount Zion while she went to see dad at Kaiser a few blocks away. It was because mom decided to stay in the city that night with dad that she called me to pick up my sister.

Anyway, after mom had dropped her off, Michelle went to the Breast Care Center trying to get in to see a doctor. My sister told me, they couldn't get her in with one of her surgeons, but she saw a nurse practitioner who said everything was fine with the new expander and sent her home. Still, the pain's grip grew tighter and ferocious.

The next day, mom would try to help again. She called the Breast Care Center begging them to take another look at my sister to find some way to relieve the pain. Mark drove Michelle back into the city to deliver her to the hospital. She waited all day and into the evening, but no one would see her.

Around 8 p.m., mom left dad at Kaiser and joined Michelle at Mount Zion. After no one saw her at the Breast Care Center, they decided to take their chances at the VA. Mom drove Michelle to that hospital where they spoke with a doctor who said she needed to be hospitalized. The VA doctor called Mount Zion and got her admitted that night.

Michelle was hooked up to a machine that fed an hourly dose of 1.5 mg of Dilaudid into her body. Unfortunately, her body had built up a resistance to the pain medications. After all, she had been taking upward of 16 mg of Dilaudid every hour; the hospital's solution wouldn't dent the pain.

She tried explaining this to the hospital staff, but nothing changed. At least not until, as she said, she lost it. She went out into the hallway and began screaming until someone would help.

Long after this incident, Michelle said, that's when they responded to her pain by loading her up with a cocktail of Methadone and Norco. Methadone is a strong pain medicine and also the alternative detoxification medication they offer heroin addicts to wean them off the drug. I hope that gives a clearer idea of how much pain she was in. Looking back, I wish I had understood better at the time.

Throughout the process, mom was terrified Michelle was becoming a dope addict. As soon as she could stand it, Michelle told the hospital to wean her from the heavy-duty medicines and decrease the dosages until she could rely on something milder.

In the years that followed, even though her body is never absent pain, she tried to stay away from powerful drugs in preparation of the day's arrival when she requires the numbing medication. The day when she finds out another cancer is attacking her body.

While getting her pain under control that week, the hospital pumped her full of medicine that would kill any infection developing in the breast expander.

She would end up spending a week in the hospital, but they nearly kicked her out early.

A few days into her stay, and while she was completely stoned on the hospital's legal drugs, a male nurse came into the room and told her to pack up and leave. She was still in terrible pain and she said she couldn't administer intravenous antibiotics at home. She called mom. Michelle was panicked, crying. Once again, mom came to the rescue to protect her family. She called the hospital, worked her magic and got them to hang onto Michelle longer (and keep that male nurse away from her).

By the time she was released, she had been weaned off the worst of the painkillers, and they cleared out the expander infection that was causing the intense pain.

Michelle wasn't the only person the hospital wanted to kick out that week. She told me about a woman who had a mastectomy. When they said it was time she should leave, the woman protested in fear.

"She just couldn't handle it. She didn't want to leave the hospital. They got the police and dragged her out of there. She was in tears and everything," Michelle explained. By that weekend, Michelle was one of the only women left in the ward. "They kicked out everybody to make room for the new batch.

"It was an assembly line. You were a piece of shit to come in, get your breast hacked off, and get thrown out as soon as possible. They didn't care if you got complications; that's your problem," Michelle said.

While my sister was getting help at Mount Zion hospital, mom was also dealing with dad's health. She had been visiting with Michelle when she received a call from a doctor at Kaiser a few blocks away. She was told to get to the hospital right away.

She ran down the street to Kaiser and up to dad's room where she found some nurses and three doctors standing around dad's bed. Dad was laying there unconscious with his mouth hanging open.

"Oh, shit. He died." That's what my mom said she thought when she entered the scene. "Honest to God, that was the first thing that came into my mind; he's dead," she told me later.

One of the doctors told mom, "He's in a coma and we don't think he'll come out of it."

Leave it to my mom to tell death to fuck off.

"Like hell," she told these physicians.

She went to my father's side, leaned over the bed and yelled at him, "God damn it. If Shackleton can make it, so can you!" Only a year before, my parents had taken a trip south to Antarctica where they learned about Ernest Shackleton's legendary 600-mile rowboat trip to explore the frozen wilderness during the early 1900s.

To the doctors' surprise, after mom yelled in my dad's ear, his eyes opened.

That's right. There's no need for mysterious witchcraft and vampires, or medicine, for that matter. Mom's on the case and her nagging abilities can wake the dead. Thanks, mom. Glad you're in my corner.

Just to rib his doctors after that hospital stay, every time dad went to see his heart doctor, he would wear a T-shirt mom bought for him when we saw the musical *Spamalot*. The bold white lettering against the black shirt reads, "I'm not dead yet."

Once dad woke up and began showing signs of recovery, his doctors remained adamant against proceeding to remove the blockage in his carotid artery. Likely, he wouldn't survive the dangerous surgery.

Later, dad told me what he remembered of his unconscious state. He kept seeing a black dog in his room that remained by the side of his bed. He also saw naked Asian women. He thought it was pleasant having all the naked women and the dog to keep him company, so why should he want to wake up from that scene. Maybe he *did* have a small stroke. Mom's theory behind the nude women was because it seemed most of the nurses at that San Francisco hospital were Asian.

A few blocks away, Michelle's pain returned to her general "post-cancer and bone marrow transplant" pain. As for me, I recovered from my surgery and readied for my double mastectomy in the months to come.

CHAPTER 13:
OVARIES, TUBES AND TITS...OH, MY!

After having my ovaries and tubes removed, I had to make up my mind about the type of breast reconstruction I wanted after my prophylactic bilateral mastectomy.

I wasn't being rushed by cancer, but the possibility of getting breast cancer was never very far from my thoughts. Mom never backed away from pressuring me into having the next surgery, but I knew I had to come to terms with this transformation. It was one thing to remove my ovaries: parts that no one could see. But hacking off my tits was another monster for my mind to reconcile; these parts, in clear view, help define me as a woman.

It was frustrating hear people's comments about how it wouldn't matter that much to them to lose their breasts. I didn't think so either, but those thoughts are mutated and burdensome when it's your body that must be altered for a disease that has not, or may never, strike.

During the next several months as life went on, I began hunting for answers. I spoke with women about their reconstruction choices and searched out more information about having a TRAM. I continued with my doctor appointments and tests. And I had to start planning my son's Bar Mitzvah celebration that was a year away.

A Bar Mitzvah is like a wedding without the wedding cake; it's a celebration focused on entertaining children while keeping it enjoyable for all the adults. It was a large undertaking, but it kept my creative "Martha Stewart" party-planning brain preoccupied.

When I wasn't researching party elements and finding ways to incorporate them into a memorable event for family and friends, I would research my breast reconstruction options. I'd have to stop when the fears seeped into my brain and ill feelings tangled my stomach.

One day I was convinced implants were the way to go, and the next, I was leaning toward having a TRAM. I was going to have to make a decision, but there were still so many fears and questions. I continued asking about recovery times and always got the "everyone is different" answer.

Then finally, someone gave me information I could work with.

I had sent an e-mail to one of the nurses at the Breast Care Center asking for a clearer explanation of the recovery. I knew there wasn't any single correct answer, but surely, with the number of women who had been through a TRAM, they must have developed an approximate timeline of the recovery; a pattern of sorts.

She started with the typical caveat that recovery varies broadly among women who have had a TRAM, but then she offered information I could sink my teeth into. Here's what she wrote:

I usually divide the recovery process into week-long increments (give or take a few days). The first week, you will be in the hospital and it will be one of those weeks in life just to get through.

Initially, you will have an epidural (pain medicine into the epidural space surrounding your spinal cord) and you will gradually transition to oral pain medication and possibly a continuous pain relief patch.

The second week after surgery will be your first week at home—also a challenging one. The most comfortable position for you to be in will be with both your back and legs elevated—think of a Barcalounger (a great thing to borrow for your recovery period). You will be able to get up to walk to the bathroom and around your house a little but will pretty much stay put throughout the day.

You will be up and walking more comfortably during the third and fourth weeks—initially just around your house a bit more and outside and around the block by the end of the fourth week. This is also the time frame when your drains will be removed which makes a positive difference in both mobility and overall comfort. Some women feel ready to drive by this time but others need a little bit more time until they feel comfortable.

Week by week, your strength will return and you will get closer to your baseline. You will wean off of pain medication and increase your exercise tolerance.

My colleague, Debby, describes the recovery process as similar to a divorce. When you first ask a friend who is going through a divorce how they are doing, the response is usually "I am okay, doing better." If you ask the same person a month later how they were doing when you first asked the question, they will likely respond that they did not realize it at the time, but they were not doing that well and that now they are doing better. It is a matter of perspective and gradual healing.

Basically, it is a long recovery time that averages around 10 to 12 weeks until you are truly feeling back to baseline. Fatigue is a major factor that can last longer than that. I hope that this helps.

I wrote back to her saying she had sufficiently scared the crap out of me. After having had epidurals during my several days of labor pains during my children's deliveries, I told her, I was sold against the TRAM. I told her how after my husband read her e-mail, he described this surgery as the worst surgery he's ever heard about. Mark noted, even open-heart surgery patients are up and walking within a few days of having their chest cracked open; and they are on less pain medications.

"Screw the tummy tuck," I wrote to her. I decided I would swim more and eat smaller portions of healthier foods. I'd live with the tummy pooch created by having babies. Stealing three months away from my children and husband sounded ridiculous just so I could have a flat belly at my son's Bar Mitzvah.

As much as I hated the idea of having something unnatural like an implant stuck in my chest, I told her the implants seemed like my best option.

So there I was, convinced to have implants that day, then changing my mind again every time I pictured my sister's gnarled breast.

This wasn't a matter of picking out what shoes to wear. I was making an immense change to my body, and I couldn't make up my mind.

It was through this process of hunting for realistic information about the TRAM recovery that I decided to start writing a blog: joeysjournal.com. I knew there must be other women who had the same questions; there must be women like me who were having troubles getting solid answers from their health care providers.

Shortly after posting the first stories about my BRCA experience, I began getting comments from other women who have had a TRAM or were facing the possibility of this procedure. They, too, were frustrated and confused by the process and reconstruction choices.

During one of my appointments, I told my breast surgeon about my confusion. Dr. Esserman asked if I had spoken with the hospital's psychiatrist. I didn't know I had that option available to me. She suggested I make an appointment with the shrink who works with a lot of women facing breast reconstruction.

The day I first met with my shrink, she began by asking if I ever considered committing suicide after having received horrible news.

"I can't say I never did (consider suicide). After my sister died, I thought, maybe if I killed myself, I could be with her. But then I thought about all the movies I would miss." No, really, I was being serious. Hey, I was only 12 years old when I thought that.

I realized I had to show her I'm not totally nuts. I added, "No, I would never do something like that. I have kids." That seemed like enough of an answer. If you're a parent, you'll fully understand the true depth of those three words, *I have kids*.

Her question about any potential plans to kill myself came quickly after her first ridiculous question, "Are you experiencing any anxiety?"

Was I experiencing anxiety? Hmm. Aside from my BRCA status? Let's see. My sister's second breast cancer diagnosis, my dad's poor health, the company my husband works for was going bankrupt....

Anxiety? Most of the time, I couldn't think about the upcoming (10-hour) surgery without my heart rate quickening and tears forming in my eyes.

If I didn't take action to cut off my tits I would likely get cancer, so basically, I felt I was fucked. Yes, I told her; I am experiencing anxiety.

I'm not sure I got much relief out of visiting with the shrink, but I continued to see her a few times (as long as my insurance would pay for the expensive service). She didn't think she could offer assistance on most of my worries and related issues. I think I experienced more relief from writing my blog.

Still, it didn't help my stress level when my diet killed the camera I used to take photos along my BRCA journey.

"NO!" I shouted as I looked down at my suddenly submerged camera. Shock quickly slipped away as I reached into the large container. I grabbed my Canon out of the goopy substance that was to be my breakfast diet shake. "No!"

What do I do? What do I do? I turned on the water, quickly rinsed off the sticky liquid, trying to remember if my camera was like those semi-waterproof watches that can get a little wet. It wasn't waterproof.

I tried turning it off and then on again to make sure I wiped away any remaining shake from the retractable lens. I dried off the lump of metal as best I could and ran upstairs to ask Mark for his advice.

"Honey, look at this." He was just getting out of the shower and drying off. I showed him the image display on the camera. "This is bad, isn't it?" There were these strange lines stretching across the screen and disrupting the foggy image.

"Turn it off. You need to turn it off," he told me. "How did this happen? What'd you do, Joey?"

I cringed as I told him the story, prefacing my tale by saying it was a friend's fault this happened.

"How could it be her fault?"

I told him about her e-mail. "She's been reading my blog. She wanted me to change my photo from Jesse's rat to a photo of me since I've already lost 20 pounds. I was standing at the counter making one of my morning diet shakes, and I saw my reflection in the brass knob on the kitchen cabinet and...."

"Wait. You were attracted by another shiny object?" My husband regularly describes me as someone who has the mind of a sea bass. I get sidetracked when something shiny like a fishing lure happens by. He grinned, huffed and shook his head.

"So, I thought I would do something creative and artistic and something that hides how lousy I look this morning. I was taking some photos and then suddenly, kerplunk! My camera fell into my shake. It was the only damn thing on the counter, and that's where it fell!" As I spoke, my husband looked at me with amazement and frustration because he knew he'd be buying me a new camera by the end of the day. And no, this truly wasn't a ploy for a top shelf Mother's Day Gift. Although, that's not a terrible idea (shhh!).

"I just put all the dishes away," he said. Yes, he did the dishes. I have such a good husband. "There wasn't a cup anywhere else in sight, and you managed to drop it into the only drink in the kitchen." Mark looked at me as though he expects things like this from his wife.

"Okay, so I'm a klutz. That's why you love me, right?" Over the years, I've associated that question with too many mishaps. And lucky me, he always finds a way to laugh at my shenanigans; more importantly, he makes *me* laugh.

It was like the time I lost my prescription sunglasses in Mexico.

Before I got on that banana blowup boat with a bunch of other tourists, I had handed my hat to my husband, but didn't think to take off my sunglasses. I'd never tried one of those banana boats, and it looked like the people out on the water were having fun. Little did I know this crazy Mexican boat driver and his buddy were going to give the American touristas a *real* ride, all the while laughing at us.

My sister had been sort of bitchy to the boat driver earlier in the day and I have a feeling he found his solution to paying her back for her rude behavior.

They dragged the banana boat out onto the ocean going faster and faster until we all began losing our grip as we straddled the craft. One more fast turn, a bump in the waves and we all went flying down into the water. So did my $300 glasses! After slamming into the salt water and regaining my composure, I noticed my sinuses have never felt as clear as they did that day. Of course, watching these snake animals and other wormy things swimming around in the water made me wonder, what swam up my nose?

Mark is used to things like this happening to me. The crazy thing is, both incidents involved a common thread (rather, a strap). If I had worn the damn camera strap, or the cord I had for the sunglasses, neither item would have been lost.

"I know this is a horrible time for this to happen, but are you mad?" I asked Mark about the camera.

He wasn't.

Several hours later, my husband and children returned from Best Buy with a bag of goodies; a new game for the Wii that I could play while recovering from my surgery, and a new Cannon PowerShot.

As Mark handed me the bag, he said, "I bought the extended warranty program because the sales guy assured me, it will cover the camera if you drop it into another shake."

Oy, such a mench!

CHAPTER 14:
TICS, TOWELS AND TOURETTE'S

While attempting to muscle through my anxieties and fears about the impending breast surgery in conjunction with planning Jesse's Bar Mitzvah, my stress level was beginning to materialize in the form of paper towel piles and other odd behavior.

As months shrank into weeks leading up to the big day, every night when my husband returned home from his stressful day at work, he'd walk into the kitchen to find mounds of used paper towels. These crumpled up paper towels, sometimes still wet from my numerous hand washings, would be sitting in stacks at our breakfast nook beside my chair where I do most of my work on the computer. More stacks would sit on the table adjacent to my computer, and yet another pile would remain on the counter next to the sink.

If I happened to be sitting at the table when he attempted to collect the towels for disposal, panic would wash over my face and I would protest. He would recoil his hand for fear I would slap it.

This is odd behavior, you say? You don't know the half of it.

Rather than being formally diagnosed by a neurologist, I have been informed casually by one of our family doctors that I have Tourette's Syndrome: a condition believed to be a particularly mild and manageable form of autism.

Not the form of Tourette's that produces uncontrollable ranting and shouting of obscenities, although, I do tend to curse too much; not because I can't control my cursing, rather because it just feels good to cuss. I love saying the word, "fuck," for instance. And yet, writing it in such a clinical fashion leaves me feeling self-conscious about my choice of words. No matter, it still feels good to say it. Try it and you'll see. Go on. Say it out loud: "Fuck. Fuck. FUCK!" Doesn't that feel better? Okay, maybe not for you, but I enjoy it.

Anyway, you may not agree after my last point, but my form of Tourette's is the twitchy kind. The kind you try to hide from classmates when you're in school because of how cruel they can be when they stare at that twitching or hear your vocal habits. And it's the kind of winks, twitches, huffing, jerking and other odd behaviors you hope your friends and co-workers never notice, or at least grow to accept as part of who you are.

One time at my job working in city government, I was really tired and a bit stressed while I sat at my desk facing the computer screen and the entryway beyond. I couldn't stop blinking to the point it leaves me with headaches. Sometimes, constant squinting and blinking results in my eyes being closed long enough that I can't see for a few moments. Don't try this when you're driving.

When I finally regained control of my eyelids and stopped scrunching my nose, I noticed my co-worker friend was standing in my doorway. His odd expression was filled with confusion and the discomfort of having caught view of something that should remain private. I was embarrassed and quickly began blushing.

"Oh, I got something in my eye." That was the safe explanation most of the time, but it doesn't explain the tensing and jerking motion in my neck.

I've heard this form of Tourette's being described as "normal behaviors gone wrong." That statement is appropriate, but doesn't take away the reaction of people who don't know what the fuck is wrong with you. Yeah, there's that word again.

I have found, my Tourette's—a condition my father and his father displayed, prior to being passed down to me and my sister—is generally most noticeably brought on by stress and lack of sleep, both of which I entertained on a regular basis prior to my surgeries. Also, Tourette's generally shows up in young or pre-teen children. Mine showed up just in time for middle school when kids were at their cruelest. Yay for me! My son's showed up right around third grade. As luck would have it, he was a popular kid and didn't have to suffer the abuse I had.

So, next time you see someone jerking their head about, blinking uncontrollably, rolling their eyes back as they forcefully close their eyelids, twitching their nose, tensing their limbs, forcing out little bursts of air through their nose or mouth, raising their eyebrows or shoulders repeatedly, and too many other little (or big) "tics" to mention...be kind. Please remember; stopping these tics is like trying to stop someone from sneezing. Forcing our body to cease its unusual actions is extremely difficult and sometimes seems rather painful; or at least as annoying as having an itch you can't scratch because your hands are tied.

Just when you thought that was bad enough, combine that with a little OCD and my bizarre life is nearly complete. (I know I'll get shit for saying life with Tourette's is bizarre, but that's how it feels in my case). I'm told this is a typical combination. In my situation, the addition of OCD helps explain the necessity of the paper towel piles. I *need* to wash my hands habitually. I use the fresh paper towels to dry my hands because I have kids. You frankly don't want to know the things they wipe on towels hanging in the kitchen.

My son's "green" solution to my paper towel problem is to assign everyone in our family their own towel hanging in the kitchen. He said we could decorate the towels with our names and then, we (really, me) won't waste as many paper towels. Such a smart kid!

Creating added stress on its own, with less than two weeks to go until my big surgery, I made the mistake of finally watching the DVD I had been given months before by the Breast Care Center. It was supposed to provide more information about the TRAM and other breast reconstruction options; it was supposed to help explain general recovery issues; so I was told.

After sending our kids out of the room so Mark and I could view the DVD, we began watching the clinical presentation of the different reconstruction options. Along with each alternative, women spoke about the option they chose; as well, there would be some clinical description of the procedures and results.

It wasn't long before I felt a bit nauseated. I tried to remain calm and approach the information as a reporter doing research for a story. If I could calmly interview grieving family members after their loved one had just died, surely I could watch this program as an educational resource. I mostly held it together, but I could hear my heart beat pounding louder and faster as the program continued.

How many other women have had to watch this video? How many times have they sat frozen in a state of panic because their breasts would soon be deformed and become atypical like these women's once beautiful, natural bodies? Can I really do this to my body? I don't have cancer. No. You can do this. You don't want cancer. Focus. Fucking focus! There might be information you need.

My husband sat on the couch watching; I worried he pictured me as one of these women. Maybe he wouldn't like my body after this procedure. He said he was okay with it and just wanted me to be healthy; but what if he couldn't look at me or touch me again after this shitty procedure?

It's kind of like how people say, don't let your husband watch when your child's head protrudes out of your crotch during labor, or he'll never again want to go anywhere near your vageegee as long as that image remains seared in his memory. Maybe it's the same with the breasts. Once the soft, pleasant, organic breasts are replaced by mismatched, scarred boob mounds, maybe he won't want to go near them. *Will I lose his affection? His love?*

After the reconstruction options had been discussed, the program transitioned into something more terrifying as it offered a clearer view at these women's chests.

In slideshow fashion, one after another, the program showed the shirtless women standing in front of a plain background; their faces were kept out of view. The focus was on their chest and clearly displayed all their red, knotty scars; deformities produced by the various surgeries the women had endured. *No. No.* It was like watching a lineup of women who had survived Dr. Josef Mengele's Holocaust torture chamber.

My heart raced; I couldn't breathe. *No. No. No.* In my growing panic, I envisioned I was standing there among these faceless women who had become slabs of meat; survivors of these barbaric surgical methods. *No, no.* I couldn't move. I couldn't look away. *NO! NO!* I was suffocating.

Terror took over my body, mind, emotions and I began panting with fear. I burst out crying. I cupped my hands over my mouth to muffle my cries as I ran up the stairs. I had to seek refuge away from the dreadful visions of the scars and mangled skin displayed on those women.

The quiet of my bedroom offered no escape from the images flashing through my mind. Pictures of those headless women, and my own sister's deformed breast, rushed through my head as if I were trapped inside a bad acid trip.

Mark came running up to our bedroom to find me curled up on the bed. I was sobbing and panting. I kept crying out, "No. No. No.

No." Mark lay beside me. He was worried; powerless against the horrific images bending my senses.

"What can I do, Joey? What do you want me to do?" He was looking into my eyes, but all I saw were those women; their mangled chests. Those women. *No, no. That's going to be me.*

"No, no, no," I echoed through my panting and howling sobs.

Jesse and Sophie had followed Mark to our room where they stood by the door. "You guys go downstairs. Mommy is going to be fine, just go downstairs, okay?" They were worried about mommy who was in the middle of a nervous breakdown. I curled up tighter and hid my face, sobbing with terror. Confusion was beating me. Panic gripped my heart. "No, no."

"What can I do, Joey?" Mark asked again with some anxiety in his voice. Through all our trials of life together, he'd never seen me like this. Never before had I been controlled and abused by my fears to this extent.

"Do you want me to call your mom?" I didn't answer through my sobbing. I just tightly grasped my pillow as though it would save me from falling off the edge of this mastectomy cliff into pain and darkness and mutilation and loss.

"I'm calling your parents," he decided.

"What's wrong? What's going on?" I heard my mother's voice over the speaker. I couldn't stop crying.

"Please, you need to talk to her," Mark told mom.

"What happened? Why is she crying?"

He told her about the DVD and what we were watching and how now, I couldn't stop crying. "Will you talk to her? She's not hearing anything I say."

I barely heard my mother's voice trying to soothe me, but she sounded so far away; her words couldn't reach me in this dark place. The screaming in my mind drowned out anything she said. *NO!* She could do nothing to calm me. I could only see the scars on those women and hear, *NO!*

"Aw, Joey. Come on, now. It's going to be okay, sweetie. You're going to get through this," mom wouldn't quit.

But no, mom. It wasn't going to be okay. Sometimes life is fucked up, and it doesn't turn out okay. Sometimes you don't have cancer, and they tell you to hack off parts of your body. "No, no, no."

And then, my dad began to speak. He wasn't soothing like my

mom; he didn't express worry like my husband. No.

He picked a fight.

"All this because of your tits? You're going to be a big baby because of a surgery?" he taunted. My nasty bastard (and I mean that lovingly), tough, Bronx boy picked a fight when I was trapped in dark thoughts! Are you kidding me? Okay, well....

"It's not your body that has to be sliced up! It's a huge surgery and...," I yelled at him.

"Then don't do anything and die," he goaded.

"Fuck you, dad. This is all your fucking fault for giving me this shitty mutation. If it weren't for your crappy genes, I wouldn't be going through this hell!"

"Good. That's better," he had succeeded at his task.

I had stopped crying and panting. I paused as I calmed down and laughed through my words, "You prick."

"Glad I could help," he said.

Everyone started to laugh. My dad knew I couldn't resist such a battle. Damn, he's skilled at this parenting shit.

So, maybe this would be a good time to visit the shrink at Mount Zion. I would see her again within a week of my surgery.

"How do you think you'll react when you see your chest for the first time?" asked my shrink about waking up after the mastectomy surgery.

I imagined there would be bumps of some kind that resembled breasts, I told her. I just didn't know what to expect once those sterile dressings were removed.

"I honestly don't know. I know there will be little I can do at that point; I'll never get my breasts back. And what about the knobby scars left on my belly from the laparoscopy when they took my ovaries? When that skin becomes my new breasts, will those scars look like oddly-positioned nipples on the sides of my tits?" I pointed to various, unbalanced positions on my breasts. "I just don't know how I'll react. I don't want to freak out." I could have rambled on about my tits for a long time if she had allowed it, but my shrink gave me "homework" that, I confess, I quickly forgot.

I was supposed to visualize, uh, something or other. I don't remember. Those days, my mind forgot anything I didn't write down. That's okay; it just felt good to talk to someone (other than my family) about what I would be facing in five days hence. She suggested I go to the cancer resource library and check out a CD that will help me relax for my surgery.

"There isn't one specific CD she's talking about," said the woman working in the resource center, "but you're free to look through this area for a CD." Shelves and shelves of cancer-related resources lay before me. "What kind of cancer do you have?" *Crap; that question.* I felt my body tense.

I hated answering that question. When most people found out I was going to have a bilateral mastectomy *by choice* to avoid my dangerously high chances of getting breast cancer since I tested positive for a genetic mutation, they generally look at me with confusion followed by the question, "Why would you choose to do that to your body if you don't have cancer? Why not just keep getting mammograms?"

So, to answer the cancer resource lady's question, I cringed slightly and almost apologetically replied, "I don't have cancer." Surely, I was unlike most of the people who utilize the resource center. I added, "I tested positive for the BRCA genetic mutation." Thankfully, that was all I had to say. There was no judging, no questioning my choice or my sanity, no looks as though I had fallen out of a tree for trusting these people to slice up my body. She didn't offer her advice, only, help.

"Oh. You'll want to look in this area." She pointed to all the books, VCR tapes and CDs on a few shelves devoted to breast cancer, and then to some other general surgery-related resources. There wasn't an area on the shelf devoted to someone in my position, and that reinforced how odd it felt to become a previvor. It made me feel out of place in this hospital devoted to curing people who have cancer.

I chose a CD: *Pre-Surgical Guided Imagery Program.* I took it home and made several attempts to listen to the CD to de-stress my mind. That is, when I wasn't snapping at the kids and wanting them to be quiet, or make their racket in another part of the house; or when the phone wasn't ringing with calls from various cousins asking how I was doing.

You're making the right decision. That was what three cousins called to tell me during a single day (mom must have called them after my mini breakdown). You'll be fine. You'll pull through and be glad you did this. They all told me what they thought I needed to hear until they asked, "How are you doing?"

"I'm pretty fucking freaking out, that's how I'm doing. I'm

terrified." What was the point in trying to hide these fears?

"Of what? The surgery?"

"Actually, it's mom who is more worried about the surgery. She doesn't like that I'll be on the table for 10 hours. But I figure, that's the least of my worries. If I don't wake up, then fuck it. I have nothing to worry about. It's the pain and long recovery time about which I'm terrified."

"Yeah, but we are fighters in our family," said my cousin Golda. "Look at your dad. He should've been dead 20 years ago." I laughed. She was right. Regardless of the diabetes that regularly finds new ways to steal my dad's youth and vitality, he had already lived decades longer than his parents and only sister had. They all died relatively young, and my dad would be turning 80 the month after Jesse's Bar Mitzvah.

Still, it was easy for someone else to say I would be fine. They weren't the ones who would have an epidural for several days after surgery. They wouldn't have a tube loaded with an abundance of narcotics stuck in their back that would be there to help me maintain a loopy state of mind (I hoped). They weren't the ones who would have to get themselves out of bed for the first time and hold a pillow against a belly with a raw, healing incision stretching from one hip to the other.

I know they meant well and were caring enough to call and want to visit, but the path I chose was one filled with anxiety, crying, depression, sadness, loneliness, confusion and anger. And just when I thought I had faced as many difficult questions as I could, my best friend asked one more.

Lilly asked, "Are you mourning for your breasts?"

I hadn't thought about it that way. That's what I told my friend whom I've known since high school. Yet, I suppose that is precisely what I had experienced when I thought about how it would feel to look down at my chest for the first time after my surgery.

If things went as planned, at least I'd have some sort of breast-like mounds without experiencing what happened to my sister's breast with the infections and being left with half a flat chest for so long while her body healed. That unnatural vision of her mutilated "raw hamburger meat" skin left me with fear and terror of what could happen to me.

I'm crazy to do this procedure, my brain screamed at me on a regular basis as some sort of instinctive survival mechanism kicked in. But then logic struck every time I looked at the faces of my children.

I have to do this, if only for my babies. I have to do this so I can see them grow and reach their own milestones. I wanted to be around for their first dates, proms, graduations, college, love, successes, weddings. I wanted to be around when they fall and need help; when they suffer and need support. I wanted to be there for them like my parents have been here for me whenever I needed them.

When this all began that August day when I heard the test results, the people around me said it's better to know so I can clearly choose my path and protect my body from the ravages of cancer. I realize it is better to know, but I really hate knowing about this homicidal mutation. I didn't want to take the test for many years because I was afraid of how this knowledge would affect my life and the people I love. After the truth was revealed at the end of that summer, this knowledge created hell in my mind; a hell that became increasingly unbearable.

From the time I was given the test results, breast cancer became the first thing I thought about when I woke up, and the last thing that drifted through my mind when I closed my eyes at night. I was tired of thinking about it. I was tired of fearfully pondering, is this the day I find out I have breast cancer?

It was like after my eldest sister died. Over the years, the agony of her death might have become more manageable, but that pain never went away; you don't simply get over something like that. There's not a day that goes by that Renee doesn't enter my thoughts. These past two years when I needed her most to face this surgery, she wasn't here to offer the comfort only she was able to provide. The comfort I remember fondly and vividly as though she walked out the door yesterday. And yes, I have another sister, but after all the shit she's gone through with her cancers, I refused to burden her with my crap as she started her life over again.

After that Tuesday in May, after this mutation will have stolen my tits, my chances of getting this cancer would drop to almost nothing. *Almost* nothing. I still have to be screened every year; there will be MRI scans, doctor visits, blood tests. Semiannually, I must have a gynecological exam. As well, every six months, my blood will be drawn for a test called CA-125 to see if some chemical levels are unusually high; I remain at risk of peritoneal cancer, which resembles ovarian cancer, and appears as difficult to detect.

It will never leave my mind that cancer surreptitiously strategizes to ambush my body, and I despise that knowledge. My guard will forever remain fortified, fueled by fear of pain and chemo and suffering and too many lasting side effects: aching body, sharp pains striking out of nowhere, sensitive teeth, shingles, less strength, back pain, ongoing hot flashes, and numerous side effects my sister is forced to muscle through.

So, back to this CD I was supposed to listen to; the one that was supposed to take the edge off of all the monstrous visions in my head and quiet the ongoing bombardment of questions filling my mind. Questions that included things like, what will that new skin feel like? My sister said it feels numb.

I began running my hand along the skin of my breasts, over my nipples, in an attempt to lock that sensation into my memory. I wanted to remember how it felt as the slightest touch carried tingling pleasure to my brain. Would I remember that sensation? Too soon, would the day arrive when I couldn't remember, and I would emotionally crumble? Will it be just like the day I ran home crying to my mom because I could no longer hear my dead sister's voice? Her laugh? I felt I had betrayed my sister's memory when I couldn't remember those things. Will I feel like less of a woman when I lose these physical possessions—these breasts—that have brought pleasure, or have fed my children?

Shit! Listen to the fucking CD!

The recording began with a woman trying as best she can with her most calm, soothing voice to explain the benefits of guided imagery and how it is supposed to help speed up recovery. She suggests the listener may want to use headphones during the surgery with this CD playing. Actually, her "soothing" voice became rather annoying by that point.

But finally, something she said did make me begin imagining a scene, except it didn't provide the calming response the voice was shooting for. Rather, the woman's soothing speech made me laugh out loud.

"...And because this method deliberately encourages this dreamy mind state, please don't play it while driving."

Really?

CHAPTER 15:
PLANNED MAINTENANCE

You know how periodically, websites go offline to carry out "planned maintenance" for an hour or two. That's what it felt like my body was about to do. My conscious mind would be shut down for about 10 hours while two surgeons and countless support staff worked on my body like a piece of meat until I had my breasts removed and replaced with skin and tissue stolen from my belly before waking up with, as websites call them, new skin; a new overall appearance.

Once again, I drove into San Francisco for a pre-op appointment. I was called into the back offices.

"You're having a TRAM Flap? I watched one of those surgeries the other day. It's a really cool procedure," a young man in blue scrubs said as though he was talking about some new shoot-'em-up action film.

"Yeah, uh, not when you're the one they're doing it to," I told this UCSF medical guy as he took my vitals (temperature, blood pressure, oxygen level, weight, and so on).

I added, "I watched it, too." He looked confused. "I saw the procedure on YouTube," I said as I stood on the massive doctor's-office scale that always weighs me at least four pounds heavier than every other scale. I've actually asked them to zero the damn thing before weighing me, but that makes no difference. After having lost more than 20 pounds in preparation of this surgery, those extra pounds make an enormous difference in the mind.

After telling him about the graphic nature of the YouTube video (do a search and watch it if you have the guts—no pun intended), this young guy must have believed I was mentally

140

prepared for these doctors to butcher large sections of my body. More likely, he was an inexperienced idiot because suddenly he thought we were ol' chums shootin' the breeze about my impending slaughterfest.

All I could think was, *shut up. Shut up. SHUT UP! What I'm about to do isn't "cool." It's necessary and barbaric. And with my luck, the day after I have my tits sliced off, some genetic jock will announce she's developed a shot to be given in the left buttocks that can alter my mutated gene and prevent the same breast cancer from taking hold of my body just as it has already killed or tortured too many women in my family. SHUT UP, you little shit!*

Good thing this kid didn't try to have this conversation with me a few months before when I would begin sobbing at the very mention of my surgeries. I might have ruined his cheery fucking morning.

After he had finished measuring my now-raised blood pressure, we began walking down the hall toward the exam rooms. Before I got very far, he stopped me and said, "Actually, we're going down *this* hallway." He directed me toward a closed door at the end of another short, darkened passageway.

As he opened the door and led me down the quiet corridor past various offices, my stomach tied in knots. "We're in here? Where they do the genetic counseling?"

"Yup, this is the place." This guy was too damn jolly to be working with people like me who have this mutation, or worse, with all the people who come to this place to deal with the most catastrophic health crisis they've ever had to battle.

"I hate this hallway," I muttered. We walked by a few offices before he showed me the room in which I would have my appointment. The room with a shitty view.

"Here you go," he said with more of his damn enthusiasm.

"This is Beth Crawford's office," I said, pausing in the doorway, one hand grasping hold of the door jamb as if I were securing my safety during an earthquake.

"Yes. It is," said the happy little fucker.

"Great," I faked. "This is where this all began."

This pisher finally gets it. (Pisher is yiddish for young, inexperienced shmuck. Oh, wait, that's more yiddish. Shmuck. Do I really need to explain that one? Well, maybe not a shmuck exactly, but childish.) It appeared to sink in that I was not exactly relaxed.

"Oh, uh, if you feel more comfortable, I might be able to move you to...."

"No, that's okay." No. Of all the offices in this place, why not leave me Beth's office, you little shit. The headache I'd battled from the moment I opened my eyes that morning began throbbing. My stomach felt sour.

The pisher left me and closed the door. The pre-op nurse would arrive any minute. That gave me just enough time to think, think, think, think, think. Oh joy. I looked around the room and mostly it looked the same as the first time I was there. Three standard chairs and the black ergonomic office chair in front of a desk that still displayed no evidence of a personal touch. There were no photos of children or loved ones, no special drawings, no photos from memorable trips. Nothing in that room would relieve Beth's stress level after telling someone they have the gene mutation, and they are about to enter hell.

I sat in the same chair as last time. Next to the window looking out over Divisadero Street. I looked around the room.

Next to Beth's desk sat stacks of the genetic testing kits. "BRCA Analysis: Discover the Risks - Understand the Options" was printed on the box that would sometime soon hold the blood test of some other genetic mutation cancer target.

Up on the window sill, sitting against the wall sat a box of sterile gloves. And there was a small box of standard hospital-issued scratchy tissues: a poor choice for people like me.

There was a display of business cards: internal medicine doctors, genetic counselors, and a card listing ovarian cancer symptoms.

While waiting for the nurse to arrive, I took notice of several cancer-related resource pamphlets: *Cancer Resource Center: Supporting wellness and the healing process, Breast Cancer Prevention Program, Donating Tissue for Medical Research*.

I wondered, *do you have to be alive or dead to donate that tissue for research*. Dying. Certainly, it's a possibility, especially in my family's surgical playbook.

Only three days before my surgery, the question arose of what to do with my body; just in case. There's always a "just in case."

Whether I wanted to face it or not, there was always that chance I could die on the table during those 10 hours, or later from complications following the surgery.

I'm not just trying to be my sweet pessimistic self; these outcomes *do* happen. That's why my parents met us for dinner at a small Mediterranean café. Dad brought me a form to fill out for the hospital regarding my health care decisions, and then they would join us for Shabbat services at our synagogue.

If I became unable, I wanted the people around me to make decisions about what to do with me. Heading into surgery, there's one outcome that is fantastic, and too many alternatives that are not. Other than the single fabulous scenario of everything going well with as little residual pain as possible, my paranoia-poster-child brain said I should prepare for anything.

Death is one obvious outcome. But in my opinion, if my brain died and my body continued living supported by machines, that would be worse than death. I wouldn't want to live like that. It would be too painful for everyone around me. Not to mention the draining expense on my already stressed-to-the-max husband. It's selfish and cruel and unnecessary.

Therefore, I told my family, "If I should die, I want to give my useful parts to people who really could use them." I preferred being used for transplants. I didn't want end up as some first-year med student's chop-job dissection project or, for that matter, to rot in some open grave with the CSI guys studying the decomposition of my body.

Then, I added, bury the remainder of my body in a simple pine box. I want to be in that pretty cemetery where our family's close friend "Hotdog" Mike was buried a few years ago after his cancer took his life. I certainly don't want to be buried in that cold cemetery where the rest of the family is; and I don't want one of those fancy coffins.

"Why wouldn't you want to be with the family?" mom asked.

Why? I certainly don't want to leave my heart in shitty South San Francisco.

"You think I want to be stuck in that cold, crappy place with its year-round fog?" We moved away from that horrible area a long time ago, and I certainly don't want to move back; dead or alive.

After moving to the warmer climate in Marin, it took several weeks of my mother trying to convince me that I didn't need to carry a parka when I played outside. "I know the fog is going to roll in, mom," I would tell her. It would be in the 80s outside while I continued wearing that heavy blue parka with the bright red lining. I certainly don't want to endure cold days and nights in that crowded cemetery in South City.

"But you won't have anyone to talk to," mom said. Yes, my mother is talking about how I may become lonely after I die.

"Precisely! You think I want to be listening to a bunch of whining and kvetching Jews for all of eternity? 'Oy, my back hurts, my skin feels so dry, my children never call or visit.' Ech!" I answered my mother, mimicking our relatives.

"I'd rather be where it's warm; where there are pretty trees and rolling hills covered in summer grass that ebbs and flows with a soft breeze. And Mike will be there. He's fun to talk to. Put me there, or out by the coast where I can sit on the beach and watch the waves crashing on the shore." Yes, these are real conversations and not just made up in my head.

I probably should not have completed this form at the dinner table with the kids sitting there (bad mommy. Bad mommy!), but I had my retired-attorney, going-blind-from-diabetes father there and I wanted to make sure I was filling it out correctly. I frankly didn't want to end up as someone's science experiment.

"If I am dying, it is important for me to be: At home. In the hospital," I read out loud.

"Is mommy dying? I don't want her to die," whined my youngest.

"No, sweetie. Mommy isn't going to die. They just want all the bad information; but they will do everything to keep mommy alive so she can come home to you and your brother," mom told her.

"I want mommy to die at home," she chimed back as if she were choosing between going roller skating or to Chuck E. Cheese.

"Nah, I'd rather die in the hospital. It's more difficult to sell a house after someone has died in it," I responded.

"Yeah, you're right," said mom, a former realtor.

And anyway, you expect people to die in a hospital. It's just creepy to think of dying at home. I remember that sickly sweet smell that stuck around the house for a long time after our Saint Bernard died when I was a kid. Yuck. Don't want that in my house.

Everything was filled out and witnessed by the waitress and her friend, and off to synagogue we went. There were going to be some speakers discussing elder care facilities in Sonoma County and how to avoid senior citizen scams. I thought my parents might be interested to hear what they had to say.

In case I haven't mentioned it before, I consider myself more of a "cultural" Jew rather than a "religious" Jew. Consequently, it may seem strange to find me in synagogue celebrating Shabbat. In fact, during the six years since we had joined this conservative synagogue, we had only attended one other Friday night Shabbat service; and that was a week prior.

We have been to High Holy Day services and numerous holiday celebrations; many of which I helped plan as part of the religious school parents' committee. I was raised under reformed Judaism, but I wanted my kids to attend a religious school that offered more than what I had experienced. I thought they should receive a foundation of Jewish knowledge, culture and experience. Then, when they grow into adults, they can decide on their own what they want to do with regard to religion.

That first Shabbat service we attended the week before was the monthly "children's service." The rabbi gets all the kids involved with the service by saying the Hebrew prayers they've been learning in class. There's a dinner, the service, then dancing and treats. Jesse's teacher, who was from Israel, sang Hebrew songs with the band.

We had missed all the other children's services, but because Jesse was expected to attend a lot of Shabbat services that year leading up to his Bar Mitzvah, we needed to go anyway.

We arrived about 15 minutes early. With only two cars in the parking lot, the kids were convinced we had the wrong night.

"No, sweetie. It's Friday night. It's Shabbat."

Sophie went running ahead into the courtyard and through the social hall and sanctuary before running back to us and yelling, "He's here! That guy is here!"

"That guy? You mean, the rabbi?" I asked.

"Yeah, that rabbi guy," she called out. I'm such a terrible Jewish mother.

Seeing me walk in for a second week in a row must have been a shocker for the rabbi. He looked nearly as surprised as he had the week prior.

"I bet you didn't think you'd see us here again tonight," I said to him. He was at a loss for words. My mother crashed the conversation.

"So, I hear we're related," she said to him. That's right mom, make the guy feel bad. Remind him how he is distantly related by marriage to the member of his synagogue who has issues with God.

"We've probably passed you at various family events," she added with enthusiasm.

The rabbi kept trying to escape our conversation because people were arriving for the service and he needed to get ready in the sanctuary. Mom continued talking as much as she generally does until he finally found a safe break and raced away.

Over the years, I've had a number of interactions with our rabbi, but mostly in regard to our children attending the religious school.

Most of my life (ah, who am I kidding…all of my life), I have felt like a misfit. And yet, something changed when I stood in the synagogue's sanctuary during that first Shabbat service the week before. After speaking with the rabbi and some new friends who entered my life because of my impending surgery, for the first time, I felt I had a community.

That feeling is tremendously empowering.

The synergy of my friends from the synagogue combined with friendships developed through my children's schools created a circle of support that allowed me to breathe.

No, this wasn't some spiritual moment of enlightenment. Simply knowing I had this support system in place allowed me to approach my surgery with greater calm and one less thing to worry about during recovery.

Don't think I'm going all weak in the knees over religion. Even the rabbi didn't expect me to become spiritual when I requested he send out a "Caring Community" e-mail to the members of our synagogue. The synagogue sends out those e-mails when there's a celebration, a birth, a death, or even when someone has surgery and they may need positive thoughts or assistance during their recovery process.

"They don't have to pray to anyone; I'm just asking people to put good thoughts out into the universe on Tuesday when I'm on the table. I figure it can't hurt," I told the rabbi.

It could be like when my sister had her first breast cancer. Everyone had ideas for bringing positive energy around her to help her heal, I explained. "One of my mom's Chinese friends told her to put red ribbons on the furniture throughout the house. She said the powerful color would bring good luck. Suddenly, my mom was hanging red ribbons everywhere." Some of the ribbons remained attached to furniture in mom's house years after Michelle's first cancer.

"Actually, that's Kabbalah," said the rabbi.

"Really? What do ya know," I was surprised.

"Well, don't worry. We'll get the word out, and you'll have more meals and help than you can possibly need," he said. He also agreed, based on our past conversations, it's probably better we leave God out of it. I found his acknowledgement of my "issues with God" and his unconditional caring to be immensely comforting. In that moment, I realized it is okay I feel like such a fuckup in too many ways.

It's okay that I don't practice the religion of my ancestors as respectfully as I probably should. It's okay to approach the rabbi and ask for help. It's even okay that during Shabbat services while looking down at the prayer book and trying to follow along with the transliteration of a Hebrew prayer, we didn't notice everyone stood up near the end of that prayer.

Everyone was standing except for my family. Making matters worse, we were in clear view of the rabbi and everyone attending that night. Then, of course, there was Sophie's behavior. After everyone would sound an "amen" at the end of various prayers, my daughter would call out a lone, "Yay!" Regardless of our religious flaws, the rabbi still found it in his heart to leave the sanctuary during the silent prayer and return with Tootsie Rolls to offer to my children.

So perhaps in keeping with my theory of organized chaos, I was sent to test the rabbi's patience when dealing with someone who may question God and faith. Maybe this genetic mutation and resulting surgeries were the universe's way of challenging my sense of control by producing an ironic necessity.

What I mean by that is the following: Since the time my children were in pre-school, I (or my husband) have always insisted on driving our kids on field trips. This ongoing rule is a result of having lost my sister when she was killed as a passenger in a car. It's taken years of knowing some friends to allow them to drive my children anywhere, even down the street. Moreover, I have turned down many offers of carpooling because of the control I maintained over what cars in which my children were allowed to ride.

Already, I experience anxiety when my children are passengers in mom's car, or even in my own husband's car. But as we approached summer vacation I had to find a solution to transporting our children to all their activities. I find it ironic that one of my greatest needs was to trust others to drive my kids during my long recovery.

A friend pointed this out to me. Yes, it is truly ironic. So, maybe someone or something truly *is* trying to send me a message.

CHAPTER 16:
MOTHER'S DAY ON THE ROCKS

When I woke up on Mother's Day, the final countdown to Tuesday's surgery had begun. In order to keep my mind off the big day, my husband kept me on the rocks all day. Yes, with two days left before my surgery, he and the kids planned a day with cards, gifts, chocolate (my favorite, See's dark chocolate), Alcatraz, dinner out and seeing the new *Star Trek* movie. Phew! That's a lot to fit into one day; which is good when you're trying to forget about your tits getting hacked off.

The morning began with cards (including one from our bitchy cat Lucy who hated me and adored Mark) and gifts; I love homemade gifts and cards from my children. One of my favorite parts of being a mom is receiving my children's handmade treasures. I save them all.

Following the "Happy Birthday" tune, Mark and my children sang, "Happy Mother's Day to you, happy Mother's Day to you...." I watched them carry all their gifts to me as I woke up to their happy faces. I opened my presents and Mark had us get dressed and ready to go.

"It's going to be cold, mommy," said my youngest. With that, I figured out where we would be going. Alcatraz Island. That's right, my husband was taking me to prison on Mother's Day.

"I haven't been there since I was a kid," I told my family. "You know, the only time locals go is because someone comes into town." It's like walking across the Golden Gate Bridge or going Fisherman's Wharf. The last time I went to Alcatraz was when some cousin was here from back East; Ohio or Michigan.

When my cousin was here in the early 1980s, I remember my

149

dad driving through the Castro District just to instill a little culture shock in this small-town teen; give him a souvenir story to bring home to the folks. When we passed two guys standing on the sidewalk and kissing, my cousin didn't know what to do. As we sat in the back of my parent's station wagon, he leaned over to me and told me what he had just seen.

"I think I just saw two guys kissing," he wasn't sure if he believed his own eyes.

"Yeah. So, what?" I had to chuckle. It was no big deal for me having grown up in the area.

Alcatraz was fun. The kids enjoyed the short ferry ride over to the island, and it was a perfect day to be out on the bay. The clear, sunny day offered some warmth against the cold breezes gusting across the water.

When we first arrived, there was a ranger gathering everyone together at one of the buildings at the bottom of the hill. He asked some people where they were from. We could hear various languages spoken in the crowd. Then he asked Sophie where we were from. She kept quiet (for the first time in her life) and looked up at me.

"Oh, we're from here," I told him our city.

"Well, you're right across the bay. Who's visiting from out of town?" he assumed.

"This is my Mother's Day treat."

"Oh," he had an odd expression on his face as if he wanted to ask, why the hell were we at Alcatraz?

We walked around the island, otherwise known as "The Rock." We strolled up the steeply-graded road to the top of the hill where the jail cells are housed. Too many times, Mark talked about how he thought I hated being there.

"No, I'm having fun. I haven't been here in so long." There was one thing I did miss. When I was here as a teen, they used to do the tours guided by rangers; some of them were former guards at the prison. They would all have their little stories filled with individual details. Now, the excursion is an audio tour with everyone walking around wearing headsets. That was a bit odd, but with the large crowds of visitors, I suppose it makes more financial sense.

It was a fun afternoon. It mostly kept my mind off the surgery except when I looked out at the view of the city and thought I caught a glimpse of Mount Zion Hospital where I would be residing in a couple days.

Otherwise, there were the creepy places to see, like the morgue that was stinky, and the timeworn buildings constructed during the Civil War. We even saw a pair of exhibitionist seagulls screwing next to where everyone waited in line for the return ferry.

"Mommy, what are they doing?" asked Sophie.

"That bird is giving the other bird a piggy-back ride," I told her.

Back on the mainland, after returning to the car, we changed into our stylish dinner wear. Yes, I changed into another outfit in the back seat or our car. Why not? The windows are tinted. I got used to doing that in our younger days when we would go up to Tahoe for the day and ski from the first lift up the mountain, to the last run of the day. We'd hike back to our car loaded down with all our ski gear, and I'd change out of my ski pants and layers of clothing in the car as Mark drove down the mountain.

"You clean up well," said my dad at our next stop after he found out I changed in the car. My parents met us in the city for an early dinner at one of our favorite restaurants, The House of Prime Rib. What? Did you think someone would actually cook dinner? Not in my family.

We're not big drinkers in my family and that night, I was the only one having any alcohol to drink: a Ravenswood Zinfandel. Yum! I ordered it after hearing one of mom's comments.

I wasn't thinking about the surgery at all until mom said, "I hope your aunt remembers she's flying in tomorrow."

Thanks for that, mom. My worries returned, I tensed up and needed that drink. With Donna's arrival, it meant I would be only hours away from my surgery since she was helping us the first week.

Donna was excited about the opportunity to organize my house when she wasn't caring for our children, and I was exceedingly glad to have her help. Mom's idea of organizing is to throw everything into the garbage; that meant anything left on the kitchen counter—such as bills, report cards, or whatever—was swept into a garden bag and tossed out. Thank heavens for my aunt's fabulous OCD organizational skills that included keeping mom away from her task.

Dinner was delicious, as always. It was pleasant sitting by the fireplace in a restaurant I have been going to since I was a child. As well, my mom, a San Francisco native, has been dining there since she was a child growing up in the Marina.

I found out later, my wonderful husband wanted to make sure we got a reservation at this popular restaurant for this particular pre-surgery Mother's Day celebration; he made the reservation a month earlier. Wow, honey...I'm impressed!

After dinner, it was time to head home, but not before stopping to watch the new *Star Trek* film at our local movie theater. That stop was spontaneous since we figured I wouldn't be healed up enough to go out to the movies before they stopped playing it in the theater.

Even though it was a Sunday evening and a school night, I didn't care if we kept Jesse and Sophie out until nearly 10 p.m. Screw it, I thought. They would be stuck in the house a lot the next several weeks.

That night, I had troubles sleeping and all I could think about were lists, lists and more lists.

I had lists by the bed, lists on the board hanging on the fridge, lists in my head. Pack this, wash that, download audio books (Dean Koontz: slipping into his imagination was just what I would need when I'm high on Morphine), spend time with the kids, oh, and take the kids to the dentist for their 6-month checkup.

Imagine that. I set up their appointment 6 months back, and it happened to fall on the day prior to my big surgery.

My parents came to the rescue again by meeting me at the pediatric dentist's office; they would take Jesse to swimming and I would wait for the dentist to finish working on Sophie. Jesse has always been easy at the dentist. Sophie, on the other hand, has been a drama queen complete with screaming, squirming, coughing, vomiting from being excessively upset, and more screaming. And all that was before they got anything in her mouth; even dental floss.

She would be paying for it now; eight cavities that had been small at the last appointment had become significantly worse by this time. She needed to return in the next few weeks at an out-of-pocket cost of nearly one grand.

"What? You've got to be kidding," my mother bitched. "Just wait until you feel better before you take on anything else."

"That's why I need to know if you can take her," I said.

"Does she have to do it now?" mom asked the woman behind the desk who was trying to schedule the appointment. "My daughter is going in for major surgery tomorrow. And anyway, what's the use of fixing teeth that are going to fall out soon enough?"

Another woman in the office walked away and returned with the dentist.

"It can wait a few weeks," she explained to mom before adding, the cavities would only get worse. As well, she wouldn't conduct the 2-hour procedure that involves laughing gas and numbing shots if it were on teeth that would be falling out soon; she would still have some of these teeth when she was 13 years old.

"Well, you shouldn't be doing this now," my mother insisted.

I added this task to the growing lists in my head, but I couldn't fight the wave of emotion that came over me when I said, "But I need to have this settled before I go in tomorrow. I don't want," I couldn't finish my sentence through tears. "I don't want her to be in pain. I just need to know this appointment is in place. I'm the one who takes care of these things."

Another office lady handed me a box of Kleenex.

"I'm sorry. I've managed to hold it together until now, and I'm sorry." I felt stupid crying in my children's dentist's office.

"No, don't be. It's okay if you call us later."

I didn't want to wait. I set up the appointment for three weeks later. I couldn't stop thinking about how I need to be around for my kids. *No, think of the lists. The fucking lists will keep your mind occupied so your stomach doesn't feel sick and your head won't hurt. Lists, damn it! What do you need to do today?*

I pulled myself together and made the appointment. My mother reacted as if I were crazy. *No, mom; you're not going to foul up my relationship with a doctor my kids have been seeing for years; a doctor who puts up with all of Sophie's dramatic crap.*

We finally left and returned to the house for a while before going to dinner. On my list, I had wanted to cut some roses to put in the house; to put in the guest room for my aunt. My mom offered to help. *Okay, let her do it.* After all, she always makes beautiful arrangements for her home.

I gave her a large wicker basket in which to carry any clippings, and she set out into our yard. Unfortunately, because most of my roses were too tightly closed in buds or spent after blooming the week before, the yard's pickings were slim. Therefore, mom cut off the flowering branch of a bush in our back yard. She brought it in and placed it on my counter. The small yellow flowers had a foul odor and as soon as she set down the clipping, I noticed numerous tiny insects spreading out and racing away from the branch.

"Mom, bugs are going everywhere! Oh, shit! They are so tiny they're hard to squish!"

"Oh, don't worry. I'll wash them off." That didn't work. She continued her efforts to rinse the bugs away while I frantically chased after the scattering insects. She grabbed the basket that held more of these bug branches; they covered a few roses hidden underneath (temporarily, sans insects). She set the basket down on the floor.

"Mom! Now they're going all over the floor!"

"Oh, shit. You're just neurotic," she yelled.

"No I'm not! You're always complaining about the cleanliness of my house and then you bring a shitload of insects into my kitchen and let them scatter all over the place where I prepare meals!" I complained as I chased down more tiny bugs.

"Well, then why did you ask for my help?"

"I didn't. You said you would make a nice arrangement, but I don't want all these fucking bugs in my house!" I called for Jesse and asked him to kill more bugs. Sophie followed her brother into the kitchen after hearing the commotion. At the sight of the bugs on the floor, my daughter began screaming and pouncing on the insects.

Eventually, dripping water and bugs on my carpet all the way from the kitchen and through my house, mom carried the infested branches out to the back yard. She shoved the branch in a bucket and returned to the kitchen to finish her task.

Finally, she entered the dining room carrying a crappy little bouquet of flowers and placed it on the table. Years before, mom had a business making gorgeous floral designs for weddings; this poor excuse for an arrangement reflected none of her creative skill. She joined my dad in the living room.

While I was finishing up some ironing, I heard her say she was staying at our house until her sister arrived. (Yes, I was ironing. I know it was ridiculous, but I wanted my daughter's clothes to look neat in case Mark wouldn't iron her clothes after I was "gone.")

"But they aren't going to be here until after 11 o'clock," I complained. I certainly wasn't looking forward to any more of my mother's "help" that evening. I couldn't deal with any more stress, and I just wanted to spend some time with my kids before the next morning's surgery.

We went to dinner and thankfully, they decided to go home from there. *Phew!*

"Maybe mommy will bring home a baby," mom told my kids at dinner. "When mommies go to the hospital, it's usually because they will bring a baby home. Do you want another baby sister Jesse?"

"No! Yuck!" he replied. Regardless, it was a moot point considering the doctors took my ovaries back in October. *Thanks again for another baby reminder, mom.*

"Yeah, I'm hoping to come home with identical twins: Tit and Tat," I named my new breasts to be. Why not laugh at yourself, right?

Even while sitting at dinner, I had more lists running through my head. *Mop the kitchen, clean out the sink, make the bed, kill any remaining flower bush bugs, try not to snap at the kids, finish the lists of kids' activities for my aunt who is arriving tonight, spend more time with the kids.*

We managed to leave the restaurant and return to our car unscathed after convincing my parents they didn't have to arrive at the hospital before I was rolled into my 7:30 a.m. surgery. I suggested they could arrive around 11:30 a.m. to take Mark out to lunch since they would still have a few more hours of waiting after that.

"I love you, honey," mom said while hugging me. "Everything will work out fine."

I wanted to get out of there before I would start crying. We went home and I continued carrying out my lists. *Get packed, socks, undies, bathrobe, shoes.* The kids finished their homework and went upstairs to take showers. Sophie was singing and chatting away. Jesse was quiet.

Bedtime arrived. Sophie was tucked under her blankets and waited for a kiss goodnight. I turned out the lights in her room and sat beside her. Jesse came in as well and sat next to me.

"I love you guys so much. That's why I'm doing this tomorrow," I told them, fighting off tears when I said, "I'm going to miss you both and I'll be thinking about you all the time."

I was glad the room was dark. I didn't want them to see my sadness. "Everything will be okay. The doctors working on me are the best in their departments, and they've done this surgery many, many times. They want me to get better so I can come home to you two. Now give me a big huggy, Sophie."

Sophie propped herself up and threw her arms around me, squeezing me tightly. Her hair was still damp and smelled like

Hawaii. I drew in a deep breath locking the scent of her hair in my memory before saying, "Okay, sweetie. It's time for beddy-bye."

She returned to her reclined position and offered an affectionate smile lit up by a stream of light from the hall. "I love you, mommy," she said sweetly.

"I love you, too, my sweet baby girl." I leaned over and kissed her soft forehead and cheeks again and again.

"What about me," Jesse asked. "I want a hug, too."

"Let's go to your room, sweetie." He led the way to his room before offering a giant hug. He didn't want to let go. *Don't cry. Don't cry!*

We had continued our conversation before he climbed into bed. I told him daddy would call as soon as he had any news.

I hoped Mark's call would be good news.

"Good night, little bug. I love you."

I closed my son's bedroom door and went to my room. I lay on my bed and cried. I thought about my children and hoped my mother was right and everything would turn out fine.

I waited up for Mark to return home that night. After work, he drove down to the San Francisco Airport where he would pick up my aunt who was flying in that night; he would drive her back to our home. She would help us with the kids while I was in the hospital the first week.

I was so thankful to have her help, and I took her up on her wonderful, generous offer. It seemed silly for Mark to take time off when I was stuck in the city; I preferred to have him home that second week after I would be discharged.

After Mark and my aunt arrived at the house and we got Donna set up in the spare room, I still had some last-minute lists to complete. Also, I couldn't shut my eyes until I wrote letters to my children.

I wanted my babies to be safe in the knowledge I would return home; but what if something did go wrong? It happens. It wouldn't be me if I didn't think it could end badly. After all, any lengthy surgery is dangerous.

So, at 2:30 in the morning, I wrote the things I wanted to tell my children, just in case I did die on the table.

To Jesse, I'd want my boy to grow up holding onto his curiosity and good-natured character. Don't become cynical and cold. Do well in your studies and talk daddy into taking vacations and continue camping.

Don't rush love, but don't be afraid of it either. Be a good kisser and a kind, giving lover; the more generous you are as a lover, the more you will receive in return. Learn how to dance; girls like that.

Keep up with your music so when you are an adult, you don't look back and wish you hadn't quit. Grab hold of life and all it has to offer. Keep an open mind to new ideas and thoughts. Decorate your room however you want.

Just as daddy has always been a gentleman with me, be a gentleman with the girls; open doors for them and buy your prom date a corsage; girls like the kind they fit on their wrist like a bracelet because a pinned corsage may damage their gown.

Reach for the stars when it comes to your dreams and your future. Find a career that doesn't feel like work, but don't become a slave to your career. Periodically, remind daddy to take a day off from work, pull you and your sister out of school, and go on a picnic out at Goat Rock; just like I would do, pick out a rock to bring home and place it in the garden. Think of me standing next to you.

Watch over your sister.

To Sophie, I know my little girl will be strong and independent. Keep your spirit brightly shining. Never let someone drown out your voice or tell you that you won't succeed. Only have friends who treat you with respect and who are caring.

Someday, when you want to know how to tell if someone is "the one"—the one you want to share your life with and possibly marry—remember that you will just know.

You will be intimate with that person, and neither one of you will be able to hold each other tightly enough. Your worries will melt away, you'll see your future together, and you will just know they are the one you should be with.

Don't be afraid of exploring the world. Use common sense; if it feels wrong, find another direction. Be safe without being restricted. Make your own decisions and trust your instincts.

Remain close to your brother. You'll always have each other to lean on.

To both my children, I hope you will attend all your proms, always celebrate Halloween "mommy style," continue to be outgoing and participate in all your interests. I see Jesse swimming at the Olympics someday, and Sophie, surely you will be up on a stage singing your heart out or shining on the silver screen. Your daddy and I both love you. And whether I am here, or wherever, we'll watch over you with the help of bubby and papa.

I love you, my babies. Always be happy and never depend on "things" as much as you would on people to bring you joy. You are my treasures and the light that shines whenever my world grows dark.

After writing notes to my children, I thought about all my friends and relatives who had been offering kind words of support and encouragement.

I was thankful to have these people in my life. I was thankful for my family. I would take their thoughts with me into the operating room. I would try my best to keep their positive messages flowing through my mind as I fell asleep on that table and under the knife.

CHAPTER 17:
THE BIG SURGERY AND WEEK ONE

Day 1: Surgery. Tuesday, May 12, 2009

We arrived at Mount Zion at 6 a.m. for my scheduled 7:30 a.m. prophylactic bilateral mastectomy and TRAM Flap reconstruction surgery. "We" means me and Mark. After having told my parents not to worry about getting to the city to meet us at the hospital before I was rolled away, I was hopeful they wouldn't ignore my request.

I was concerned about mom being too tired to drive safely very early in the morning; but more selfishly, I was afraid she might add last-minute stress, or question my decision one last time before I was taken into surgery. I told my parents it was useless for them to be there that early since it was such a long surgery, but my mom would have nothing to do with that.

While waiting for this journey to begin, I took a photo of the urban landscape outside my pre-op room. The morning's early light created a warm orange glow on the buildings as the sun slowly climbed over the city.

I changed into my hospital gown and gathered my ponytail under the blue gauzy hat shaped like an oversized shower cap. I began listening to music on my Mp3 in an attempt to remain calm. Moments later, my folks entered the room.

Mom said she wanted to kiss me and say she loves me before I was taken away.

Nurses came in and made their preparations.

"Please, tell me your name and birthday," a nurse asked before installing an IV into the back of my hand.

Then, I was extremely happy to see the next person who walked through my door. It was Dr. Ng, the head of the anesthesia department.

When you go into surgery, many times, you don't know who will be your anesthesiologist until right before the procedure. A week or two prior, you may meet with someone from the department, but it seems it all comes down to whoever is written on the board that day.

Knowing Dr. Ng would be in the operating room with me was a great comfort.

I've had other surgeries under general anesthesia. But until I experienced the God-like skill of Dr. Ng, I'd had no other doctor who would heed my warning that my trachea is child-sized.

Many years prior, an anesthesiologist had informed me of that fact after another surgery when they had to size down the tube thingy a few times before settling on a manageable diameter. Prior to any future surgeries, the doctor said, I should warn other doctors about my small windpipe. When intubation was necessary, even a woman-sized tube was too large for my windpipe; they should opt for a child-sized tube.

Only a year before when I was having another surgery up in Santa Rosa, I warned the anesthesiologist of this physical limitation, but she disregarded the information. The pain in my throat that week was more painful than the surgical recovery. I should have sued the bitch, but what the hell; I lost weight that week because it hurt too much to swallow food or drink.

When I saw my rock-star anesthesiologist, it brought a big smile to my face. He'd been my anesthesiologist during the removal of my ovaries. Based on the information I had given to the nurse, he took extra care and my throat wasn't sore at all after that surgery. Seeing him was such a relief; one less thing to worry about the morning of my TRAM.

Dr. Ng has a calm, knowledgeable disposition. He took my hand in his and told me not to worry. I only felt relief knowing he was there, especially having been told he would be retiring soon.

"Please take good care of our little girl," mom said to him before he left to finalize preparations.

As I relaxed, I fanned away periodic hot flashes when I wasn't bundled under warmed blankets. The room was kept a bit chilly to prevent germs from growing.

Next to arrive was Dr. Foster. He displayed his usual relaxed confidence and asked that I stand next to the bed and expose my torso. He drew lines on my chest and belly regions creating a map for his surgical slices. It tickled as the tip of his pen dragged across my skin. Never again would I feel that sensation on my abdomen or breasts.

Mark recorded some last videos and took photos for my blog. And we all waited for the surgical staff to roll me away.

When that time finally arrived, I asked Mark if he wanted to cop one more feel before the girls were stolen from my chest. My silly husband wasted no time to jump at this opportunity. My mom took a photo of his enthusiastic smile when his hand disappeared under my hospital gown and he grabbed hold of my boob. He retrieved his hand, leaned over and gave me a kiss.

My parents kissed me, as well, and my dad said, "Okay, we'll see you later, Joey."

"Okay. I love you," I said as they rolled my bed through the door.

Some anxiety kicked in as I was rolled down the hall and through some wide doors. But simultaneously, I started to feel some relief that I was finally removing these cancer time bomb tits. As long as everything went as planned, I would come out the other side with new breasts and less worry about battling a cancer-filled destiny defined by my genetic makeup.

My bed was rolled into the operating room. It was cold in the large room with high ceilings and white walls. There were surgical staff members busy at their tasks and making final preparations.

Waiting by the table in the center of the room was Dr. Esserman. It was her task to remove my natural breasts, extracting as much potentially cancer-producing breast tissue as possible. She would prepare the cavities before Dr. Foster would use his plastic surgeon skills to reconstruct my new form.

My bed was placed parallel to the higher operating table. I was asked to sit on the edge of my bed and lean forward with my elbows on the table. Dr. Esserman positioned me as if I were playing hide-and-go-seek, resting my face down on my arms as I was prepared for the painful process of inserting the epidural in my back.

Across from me on the other side of the operating bed, Dr. Esserman leaned over me. She gently held down my arms, stroked the back of my neck and my hair like a mother comforts a child.

"What should I sing today?" She considered her options in this process that she has acted out countless times. "Oh, I know."

161

She softly sang a song from *Phantom of the Opera*. And then she asked, "Have you seen *Wicked*?"

Mom had season tickets to that year's musicals in San Francisco, and we had just seen it back in March.

"Oh, I love that play," she said and began singing songs from the musical while needles were being plunged into my back.

The needles stung my skin like I had just passed through a swarm of jellyfish. The pricks of needles filled with medicine were meant to numb my back before digging around to find the correct cavity for the epidural's resting place. It would remain there in my back for the next several days carrying a constant supply of pain medication to my body. In addition to the epidural and my hand IV, there would also be another IV placed in my neck.

I don't remember much after the epidural was installed in my back. The next several days would be accented by groggy memories resulting from my Dilaudid delirium. They gave me what I called a "happy button" I could push every 15 minutes to supply pain killers into my body through the epidural.

To my mother's surprise, I brought my computer and camera with me. The hospital offered internet access, and I thought I would post updates each day from my bed. While I succeeded in doing so, unfortunately, I had been doped on liberal amounts of pain medications. The result was I would write a word or two and fall asleep. Write a few more words and fall asleep.

Writing a few paragraphs became a long process. Uploading videos and photos was difficult. My mom, who was staying in the hospital overnight with me for several nights, got to learn some of these skills. Mom's brain typically shuts down when you try to explain how to do something on the computer, thus it was terrifically exciting for her when she learned how to resize a photograph.

I slept most of the first few days, only waking for some periodic interaction with the nurse, or to write on my blog. It turned out to be useless that I brought music and books to listen to. I didn't watch TV. I slept. Now and again, I would be fascinated by the fish swimming across my computer's screen saver. Otherwise, everything was quiet.

Day 2: Sleepy fevers and sharp pain

While my mind and body remained generally stoned, my fear of pain remained prominent.

The epidural mostly numbed my belly region, but on my chest, I had spots of sharp pain like a knife was sticking in my side. I lay on my back in the required upright position and generally, I was afraid to move my body; any movement resulted in pain shooting through my abdomen, chest, back.

It also felt like someone had strapped a belt around my chest and cinched it tightly, or as though someone was sitting on me. Coughing was not fun; even the smallest cough would send waves of pain through my torso.

Likewise, getting out of bed proved to be a painful challenge when I was encouraged to sit in a chair that second day. Mark took a video while the nurse gently coaxed me from my bed. I had to swing my legs around to the side of the bed, but this wasn't as easy as it sounds.

After the bikini cut I'd had back in the 1990s, I was better prepared to approach this first time moving into a sitting position. Those many years prior, I remember the nurse advising me to hold onto a pillow, but that does shit to get you out of a reclined position when your stomach muscles don't work.

At least after this surgery, they have you propped up most of the time as your stomach heals after the removal of a large section of skin.

Still, that didn't stop the pain caused by trying to spin my body around to the side of the bed. One needs stomach muscles to change position and mine had been moved around; re-tasked as the suppliers of blood flow to my new breasts. Anything resembling a sit-up had been removed from my physical abilities.

Complicating matters, after a mastectomy, it hurts to use your arms. I couldn't use my arms to push my body up from the bed and into a sitting position. Therefore, I was forced to find a new technique for sitting up absent stomach muscle and arm strength.

The nurse helping me was patient and supportive. "You can do it," she said with tenderness in her voice. "Grab my arm," she gently coached.

"Oh," I moaned with pain as I moved slowly. My body didn't want to cooperate to produce what is a natural motion for most people.

"Okay. Okay," I kept repeating as I maneuvered my way to sitting up on the side of the bed.

"Okay, you're doing it," said this marvelous, compassionate

nurse. "All right. Good job." She wanted me to remain in a sitting position for a few minutes. It wasn't beneficial for my body to become excessively accustomed to being in bed.

This day was also the first day Mark would get to glance at my new breasts that were individually masked by sterile gauze bandages and tape. I pulled down my hospital gown to show him the new girls. The skin circling the bandages was bruised. I worried he wouldn't react well, but I was too drugged to notice if he did.

More bandages covered the incision that created a new belly button to replace the one eliminated by the TRAM. And below that was a long strip of more bandages protecting the waistline slice that stretched from side to side.

Aside from all the bandages and IVs, these squeezy, pressure things had been placed on my legs; they were positioned below my knees and helped prevent blood clots from forming. And there were the mini-pillows shoved into my arm pits; those added comfort and reduced pressure on my chest and swollen breasts.

The little calico-covered pillows called "Comfort Pillows" were handmade by the Mira Mesa Women's Club in San Diego. They came with a little yellow note titled, "Especially for You." The note read, "A community service group is sending you this special pillow to comfort you and to let you know we care." It continued, "Please know that we care and pray you are healthy again very soon." And at the bottom, "Fighting breast cancer, one woman at a time." Their little pillows indeed made a difference in my comfort.

Those first few days while mom served as my evening advocate and slept over in the hospital on the cushioned chair that converted into a bed, she also became my social secretary. Mom is a talker and she remained on the phone most of that second day as countless relatives and friends called to check up on my progress.

When she wasn't on the phone, she found a Mexican restaurant down the street she couldn't stop raving about. She went there for lunch and dinner. She returned with some chili poppers and gave one to Mark who was visiting before heading off to work for the evening; he came in every day to stay as long as he could and give my mom a break from her babysitting duties.

After all her Mexican dining that day, I joked with her that we'd likely have some farting in the room. Add that to her snoring and the evening would be complete.

The first night, nurses came in every two hours to check my

vitals, especially since I had a high fever and my feet were swollen. Mom got up most of the time, otherwise, there was some light snoring and farting.

"I don't snore," mom insisted. "You're just imagining it."

"What's the big deal? I'm not afraid to admit that I snore; so does Mark," I responded. She continued to deny her nightly noise. Yeah, that's why the nurse brought me some ear plugs for the second night.

The nurses—such as Blanca, Ramonette and Ananda—were wonderful, caring, kind and sweet.

One nurse described me as a "model patient." I had been calm, easygoing, and cooperative; unlike many of the patients experiencing the same surgery, they said.

Adding to the excitement of this hospital ward, there were two inmates down the hall, both with two police officers on guard at both their doors.

It was time again to push my happy button. Pain meds began to drip, drip, drip into my epidural. I would continue writing the next day.

Day 3: Walking down the hallway, and an evening of hell

This was a tremendous day. I managed to get up and walk a few steps outside my door and back. Granted, I had a lot of support from my wonderful nurse Bettina and two others.

Additionally, I managed to get into a seated position with more ease.

"Remember to crunch down," the nurse said as I slowly swung around to the edge of the bed. "Did you press the button already?"

Nope. Press the happy button. I was going to need it for my walk.

Standing up was no small task, but once I was up on my feet, I remained hunched over, using the circular handrail on the IV stand for support. I leaned over the rail and moaned from the pain experienced with each slow step. The nurses didn't want me to walk too far. One nurse placed her arm around my waist and gently guided me down the corridor and back.

"You did very good," she said as we turned around and slowly traveled back to my room. Every day will get better, she told me. "The first time is always the hardest."

They walked me back to my room where she guided me into a

cushioned chair. "Aw, oh," the pain shot through my stomach and chest as I slowly sat down.

"Good job," she said. "Okay, take a deep breath. You want to press the button?" She handed me the happy button to hold onto and press. "That's your reward," she jested. Mark chuckled.

I coughed more on the third day causing sharp pains and lingering aching. My temperature had risen above 100 F. In order to prevent pneumonia, I had to start forcing air into a volumetric exerciser apparatus. I would exhale into a hose for as long as I was able to keep a ball floating in a tube.

Having to sit up so much in bed and not being able to lay flat or on my sides, my butt at my tailbone was starting to get miserably sore. If I had been thinking clearly, I would have asked for one of the air-adjustable hospital mattresses. I waited too late to ask and by then, the pain in my tailbone would end up lasting for several months.

And there were more pain issues. I knew there wasn't much more time left on my epidural; eventually, they were going to have to remove it and take away my happy button. I tried not to think about that concern too much. Because I thought they would be removing the epidural this day, I mistakenly asked my mom to stay one more night.

Mom decided to drive back to Marin that morning to check on my dad and take him to the hospital where he had to get a prescribed shot every week. She wanted to take him to lunch and stock the kitchen with some food. She hadn't planned on returning that night, but out of my fear, she reluctantly agreed.

I knew she should have stayed with dad, and I'd hate to be faced with guilt if anything had happened to him while she was in the hospital with me—her 43-year-old daughter—but sometimes, you just need your mommy.

She left for a few hours. That meant, I was on my own on this day when I tried putting other worries out of my mind.

One such worry involved facing doubts about my decision to have the TRAM reconstruction.

When I would chat with someone on the phone, as much as I appreciated their call, I found some of their comments frustrating.

I put out a request on my blog saying, since I've already cut off my tits, this isn't the time to say, "Well, I *guess* you did the right thing."

You guess? Don't offer messages of doubt, I requested. After all the months of worry about cancer, I was happy finally to be able to say the odds were now in my favor instead of weighing me down.

I invited people to make the same judgments only when they faced the same odds. Otherwise, I asked them to give the questionable comments a rest.

On this third day in the hospital, most of the time, it felt as though someone was sticking a knife in the side of my new left breast. Furthermore, periodically in my drowsy state, it seemed as though someone was pressing down on my shoulders. I would open my eyes and find nobody there. It was just the tightened muscles and skin trying to find equilibrium.

Something else I found out this day; nurses get excited when you reveal you farted. Mom didn't like that I wrote the word "farted." She had rather I said, passed gas.

While sleeping most of my day away, I began having some amusing dreams about having dinner at one of our family's favorite restaurants. I think we were at Roy's in Hawaii. Yes, in my delirium, I experienced hallucinations about eating out.

Regrettably, the day didn't turn out as delightful as all that.

I know mom is going to read this. Therefore, I need to preface what I'm about to write with the biggest "THANK YOU, MOM!" I possibly could offer my mother.

I wouldn't have been able to get through this extremely long process and crazy surgery without having known I had your support. I'm not an idiot; I knew you would help me through these brutal surgeries no matter what. I knew you were worried about me. If it were possible, I knew you would have put yourself in my position to take away the pain I experienced. I knew your heart was in the right place.

Now, mom, take a deep breath before you continue reading.

Mom, I know you didn't want to come back into the city that afternoon, and likely, you were emotionally exhausted by watching another daughter's body get sliced up. Still, upon your return that evening, I didn't need you to remind me of your extra effort any chance you got.

Even as I lay in bed, you did this while trying to hand me my heavy laptop computer so I could place it back on the bed table. Apparently, you thought I was going to outstretch my arm and take the 11-pound machine from you. Yes, I'd happily pull out my stitches and create agonizing pain and bulging hernias in my stomach so you wouldn't have to get up out of your chair. Let me explain how we arrived at this moment.

Earlier that day after mom returned from visiting with dad, my meal was brought to my room and mom made space on the table by removing the computer from the small rolling table.

"Well, maybe I'll check my e-mail while you're eating. I haven't been able to look at my e-mail in days since I've been stuck here. Joey, how do I get into my e-mail," she fussed as I tried reaching for a plastic fork just out of reach. "Joey, what do I do?"

"Mom, can I show you after I eat something?"

"Oh, crap. I just want to check my damn e-mail."

"Okay, here," I explained what to do.

"Oh, shit. I don't get it, Joey. You know how I am with these damn things. What do I do?" She sat there complaining as if she wanted me to get out of bed, sit with her, and explain how to retrieve her e-mail.

"Turn the screen to me so I can see it better." She did. I explained once, and then tried to return to my meal. I tried explaining again and again, fitting in a bite here and there. I tried opening a juice container, but the meds stole much of my strength. I attempted reaching for a straw with little success. All the while, mom sat there becoming more and more frustrated, agitated and angry because I wasn't helping her more.

"Oh, screw it," she said through an angry outburst. That's when she tried to hand the computer to me.

"Mom, what do you expect me to do?" I had no place to put the computer, let alone the strength to outstretch my arm and grab it from her.

After a pause and loud huff, she did get up out of her chair and place it on the bed table for me; an action she took in combination with her usual groaning and an "Oy." Okay, she's got bad knees and most of the time she makes those motions when rising from a chair. Her "Oy" just seemed a tad accentuated this time.

"What is the pain going to be like when they take out the epidural?" I asked a nurse who'd been in the room, rolling her eyes at my mother's behavior.

The nurse came to the side of the bed, reached over the bed table, took my hand in her warm palm, cupped it with her other hand and very seriously and quietly said, "You're going to feel your body."

I knew the full meaning of that statement. One word: childbirth. I was terrified by the potential level of pain when they would remove the epidural from my back; the epidural which kept my pain under control and kept me "looking good," as mom would say. I had to explain to mom several times how the epidural had been helping manage my pain. The pain was still there, only it was masked by the constant drip of Morphine and whatever else they shoved into the tubing.

"Yes, but you're healing," said mom.

"Yes, that's right, but I don't think it's registering in your brain *why* they are keeping this epidural shoved in my back for several days," I said. Okay, maybe that was a bit bitchy, but I was frustrated by her confusion.

She commented that she thought it was used for saline, not realizing it held a constant drip of pain killer.

"The pain isn't going to go away once they pull out the epidural." I was going to begin feeling everything they had protected me from up to that point. I truly feel sorry for those women who were the first to have this surgery when the doctors were still experimenting to determine an optimum protocol for pain management.

Although I hadn't been watching television more than a few short times all week, mom asked me to find a show to watch. I complied. The only thing on was a show she had never watched. She didn't know the story, but that didn't matter.

By this point, mom wanted to pick a fight.

"Turn it up. I can't hear it," she complained. I complied, pressing the "up" volume button on the small box that housed not only the controls for the TV, but also the valuable button to call for a nurse. "I can't hear it. Turn it up some more." I did. She still wasn't satisfied. At home, she and my dad had reached that age when the TV volume is turned up loud enough for the sound to carry into the neighbors' living rooms.

Mom was sitting with her feet up on the makeshift chair/bed to my left. The control box, wired from the wall behind me, was stretched as far as it would reach and rest on the bed beside my right hip. The volume seemed loud to me, but mom wouldn't stop complaining that she couldn't hear the sound from the small speaker. If I'd turn it any louder, it would have been blaring in my ear.

All week I'd avoided any noise, not even listening to the books or music on my Mp3. I tried to make her understand this, but she only grew more agitated.

"Fine, then I'll read my book," she sulked. A moment passed before, "Joey, aren't there any brighter lights in here? I can't see what I'm reading."

I don't know, mom. Let me get up and find one for you. "I don't know. Just look back there on…," before I could finish, she blew up at me.

"Oh, forget it! I'll just go to sleep!" She got up and turned off the dim light the nurses kept on during the night for their evening checks so they didn't have to turn on the bright fluorescent light above the bed.

"You've got to be kidding me," I said. Other than the television up on a platform by the ceiling, the room went dark. "The nurses said they want that light kept on at night," I reminded her.

"Well, what the hell do you want me to do?" She was getting more worked up as she turned the light on and began yelling at me.

"Wait! You can't do this now," I insisted. "You really need to take a step back and see what you're doing. This has got to stop!" Was that going to work to stem her perturbed mood and an escalation of impending warfare? Was she going to realize she was picking a fight with someone who could barely move? I couldn't defend myself with anything above a loud whisper because even loudly talking hurt.

My plea succeeded. She stood still staring at me for a moment before she replied.

"I'm just going to sleep." She lay down facing away from me and drew a blanket over her body.

I knew she wasn't sleeping, and aside from my racing heartbeat, I could hear her frustrated breathing. I sensed the tension surrounding her body, and her behavior made being in the room with her nearly unbearable. That didn't last long before she got up.

"You know what? I'm going home."

What you must understand is, by the time Mark came by the hospital before work that evening, I told mom she should go home. She had been getting disturbed by every little thing since returning that afternoon to spend the night. I knew she was tired and sick of being at the hospital. Still, she had said, with just enough guilt in her voice, "No, I'll stay."

Things only got worse after Mark left, and by the time of the swelling fight, it was already past 7 p.m. The later hour left me concerned she was overly tired or too upset to drive home safely that hour in the car. My worrying didn't stop her; she collected her things and left.

Okay, yes, I was a little relieved when she departed, but that didn't stop me from crying after she was gone. Not because I was alone, rather because there I was, stuck in bed, in pain, trying to make it through this horrible first week, and I needed to keep my mind positive. I felt as though she shattered all those feelings of strength and instead, filled me with anxiety and stress.

The longer I cried, the more I felt like all the negative energy of the day was draining my body's natural healing resources, creating a more difficult and longer recovery. It was a rough night filled with Morphine-induced nightmares of my mother yelling at me.

As I found out several weeks later, there was more to this story than mom just being in a foul mood.

Mom never returned to the hospital the next few days before I was to go home. Sure, it could be that she was tired of being there, but it turns out there was more on her mind that she wasn't telling me.

That day, she had taken dad for his medical appointment, but she concealed that she, too, had seen a doctor. Her doctor was concerned there might be a problem with her lungs. She was to go in for a computed tomography (CT) scan to see what was going on with her lungs. They wanted to find out why she was short of breath a lot.

She had her scan a few weeks later and found out she had three nodules on her lungs. They were too small to do anything about, and most people live with them, she was told. They would do another scan in July and another six months later to see if there were any change.

Weeks after that stressful evening in the hospital, mom and I had a chat about her lungs.

"If it grows, I might have a problem," she said, repeating the disclaimer, a lot of people have this and they live with it. "If the thing has grown (by July), then kiss my ass goodbye. The only thing they're concerned about is that I'm out of breath and tired all the time."

"So, what does that mean?" I asked.

"It means they don't know." She added it's not healthy to have

CT scans too often. "So, what do you do? It's like your father. He's been living with a blockage in his artery. There's nothing you *can* do."

At her appointment, they asked her what high school she went to because any public buildings from the 1940s and 50s had asbestos.

"Well, we all die, but I'm not dying yet, so I can drive you nuts for a few more years." Somehow, her statement reminded her of travel plans and she began discussing that topic. "I met this very nice man who was doing my breathing test and he wants me to adopt him. He's from St. Croix, and of all the islands in that area, he says St. John is the best."

"Mom. Focus. Tell me more about what they found."

"Right now, it looks like nodules."

"What the hell are nodules?"

"They're little dots; little growths."

She read the report. She had these nodules on both lungs, and they were approximately 5.5 mm.

If there were no change, nothing could be done. Even if the nodules grew larger, there was nothing to be done other than radiation. If they did surgery, likely she would die on the table. "It's a major operation and very dangerous. It's safer to leave it, so I'm going to leave it, have fun and enjoy every day of life. Period."

She explained these nodules are common. They wouldn't have known about them had she not had a heart attack scare a while back. I'm sure that was part of her stress that night in the hospital when she was concerned for her own health as well as mine. (Or, she was just tired of being at the hospital and showed it by being a bitch.)

"So, the nodules are fine. It's whether they turn into tumors. That's when you're screwed," she continued.

"How can they tell it's not cancer?"

"They said there's no mass to the nodules."

Mom's lungs became a towering "wait and see."

Looking back on that difficult night, it was simply a case of having a shitty day. Alas, while mom's short fuse was a poor disposition for someone serving as a patient's advocate, I understand, nonetheless.

Day 4: A lovely afternoon, and yet...

By the fourth day, I was getting up and walking mostly upright past my door and down the hall. Walking would help return circulation to my aching buttocks after a night of remaining in one position; moving or trying to turn over onto my side caused pain. I had a sponge bath. I even brushed my teeth.

In fact, I brushed my teeth just in time for Lilly to walk into my room bearing gifts. She brought a bouquet of gorgeous peonies she positioned next to the fragrant Star lilies mom had brought in to brighten up the room. These bouquets were lovely, but their fragrance was meant to offset the increasing stench growing on my body; I desperately needed to be showered to help wash away the foul odor of narcotics, antibiotics and more medicines filtering out through my skin and sweat.

Lilly brought bubbles I could blow if I felt playful, a silly straw to use with my standard pink plastic hospital cup, and a tasty variety of dark chocolates.

She was dressed in jeans, a white oxford shirt and a navy blue Armani blazer. As long as I had known her, my beautiful, tall blonde friend always looked stylish and put together. I, on the other hand, have been known to clean up well, but I've never made tremendous efforts to present myself in much more than casual appearance.

Lilly and I met in high school and became inseparable best friends. It never mattered how much time passed between our chats; we easily fall into conversation. We know each other's secrets, joys, fears.

When we were young, my very persuasive friend once told me how I was the only person who could tell her "no." I always knew she was much more refined than I would ever be, but she also knew I'd never bullshit her like some of the people who have passed through her life.

After a walk down the hall, Lilly brightened my spirits as we chat on about all sorts of girly and mommy stuff for more than four hours. I sat up in the big chair while she lounged on the end of my bed. It was just like we were hanging out in one of our bedrooms at our parents' homes when we were teenagers. Happy times.

And how magnificent of a friend is she? You don't find many friends who would readily offer to massage your butt cheeks because they are intensely sore. Thankfully, that's exactly what she did after finding out about my aching backside.

Absent any hesitation, she grabbed some lotion off the counter and happily offered her kindness. I don't think even my closest cousins would offer to do the same, especially after I hadn't had a proper bath for several days.

Later, when I asked her what she remembered of that day, I was surprised to hear all the details locked in her memory. She remembered pulling my hair back. She said I was mellow, but my attitude wasn't just the result of pain killers. When we spoke about the surgery and the resulting pain, she said I was taking everything in stride.

Near the end of Lilly's visit, the pain-management guy walked into my room and said it was time to pull the epidural out of my back. *Damn.*

At first, the worst part of his actions was the long line of tape being pulled off my back and stretched up over my right shoulder. I figured I'd look like a lopsided "Cha, Cha, Cha" Chia Pet when that hair grew back.

Because of the medicine I'd been taking, including the decreased dose of pain killers from the epidural by this point in my recovery, the man assured me, I shouldn't feel much. Unfortunately, that promise was short-lived.

It was time for Lilly to leave, and I needed some rest after a delightful afternoon. Unfortunately, in Joey's world, the deer always gets whacked. Within 30 minutes of the epidural's removal and Lilly's departure after our wonderful visit, the shit hit the fan.

I began feeling a burning sensation in my abdomen. I thought, maybe the catheter got backed up. Swiftly, the burning spread. Terrible cramping developed along the TRAM incision. I kept thinking about what the nurse had told me the night before. You're going to feel your body. But we'll have drugs to help you through it.

Where are the fucking drugs!

Before long, I was feeling all the pain the epidural had been masking since Tuesday. As well, I was crying and attempting to hold back the convulsive sobbing because it hurt too much to cry.

Staff was running around trying to figure out what had gone wrong; why there wasn't a back-up pain push button for me if the pills didn't take hold.

I called Mark who was on his way to the hospital. I called my mom. Mom was on the phone with the doctor trying to find out what went wrong and what they could do immediately to stop the pain. Mom is a force to be reckoned with when she uses one of her "immediately" speeches. Sort of, Mother Theresa meets Mommy Dearest who wants her way right now, damn it!

"You've got to calm down, Joey. Take deep breaths," my family tried to console me over the hospital phone and my cell phone.

"I know, but it hurts so much. It hurts so much," I cried out through flowing tears.

"Calm down, Joey, or you're going to hurt yourself," mom said. *Now do you understand why I was terrified of this day and being alone when it happened?*

After a while, the staff finally had me doped up and sleeping.

Mark was there when I woke up, and by then, my tailbone area was experiencing excruciating pain. I asked the staff for some help to roll over onto my side as a way to alleviate the buttocks pain. They would send someone into my room. The nursing staff had changed, and this male nurse stopped by to ask what I needed.

That guy called in another man, and they began aggressively yanking the sheet beneath me. Making matters worse, the second guy slapped a pillow to the side of my new left breast. He struck the area that had been plagued by that stabbing pain since the surgery.

I began crying in agony after my body had been jarred. Mark chased them out of the room before they could cause any more damage. He stood out in the hall yelling at them; they couldn't handle me so aggressively after this kind of surgery.

I was thankful he had gotten off work early that evening and was visiting with me.

I was given more drugs and dozed off into unconsciousness.

Day 5: I finally get to see my kids

The weekend had finally arrived which meant Mark could bring Jesse and Sophie to visit me in the hospital. I hadn't wanted them to see me at my worst. Moreover, it wasn't healthy for me to be around them when my incisions were fresh. Children catch and spread too many things, and I didn't want to suffer through a painful staph infection like my sister had.

I think I had too much dope in me by the time Mark and the kids arrived for their visit. I wanted to show them mommy was healing, but when I stood up too quickly, I became dizzy and nauseated by my rapid ascent. I had to reach out for the wall to steady myself.

My big walk got turned around quickly, and the drugs for the nausea knocked me out for most of the afternoon. Still, at least I got to sleep in the upgraded hospital bed. It was the computerized air mattress that changes with your shifting body. That bed, in combination with about 10 pillows, vastly improved my comfort level to help relieve my buttocks and back pain. I had the pillows arranged under my arms, between my legs, supporting a hip, behind my head, under my knee; they all had their own happy spots on my bed.

Sophie brought giant Mylar butterfly balloons for my room; and my babies got to hear me say I was on the mend. Their gentle hugs felt spectacular.

By the end of their visit, the worried looks they had displayed on their beautiful faces when they arrived transformed into impatient "can we go yet?" expressions once they began arguing over the use of a chair. It was time to go.

It was healing to see my kids and spend time with them.

Day 6: A mellow day with an Ativan twist

It was hard to believe I had nearly made it through the first week.

It was an exceptional day in the hospital when the catheter was removed. Finally, I could sit on an actual toilet; I could make a pee, and more significantly, a poop. And all in one day! The opiates and other medications, in combination with the surgery sending my intestines into shock, had stopped my bowels from moving. What's not to love about such a morning? *Where has my mind gone?*

I decided I would remain in good spirits even though the scary pain management guy had the courage to show his face in my room after the epidural fiasco.

No matter. It was a beautiful Sunday in the city, and I wasn't getting poked by needles. Mark was driving into San Francisco after dropping off the kids with my parents, and it was going to be a quiet day.

As well, a large proportion of the patients on my floor had been sent home which added to the day's peace. There were still some police officers guarding a door at the end of the hall. Boy, that would truly suck having to go through a mastectomy before being sent back to jail.

Also on this Sunday, it was the Bay to Breakers International Footrace in San Francisco. Oddly enough, this was only the second Bay to Breakers weekend in 19 years I had my television director husband home (or at least, at the hospital).

Most years, Mark had directed the show for the race. Leading up to this weekend, there would have been the extra meetings, longer hours and several weekends killed by work; but not this year. This year, the station decided not to do the show; not a surprise given the company's poor economic status at the time.

It was during those many months when the company's stock continued to plummet when Mark and I sat on pins and needles. We feared the day would arrive when he would go to work and find "out of business" signs pasted to the glass doors. I told him to remove anything of value out of his desk; just in case he couldn't get inside the building.

While the overtime pay is substantial when he directs the annual footrace, I was truly thankful he could spend the day with me. We both got to take more naps than we had in a while. We chatted, joked around and he even learned how to clean out my Jackson-Pratt (JP) drains once I returned home. I had four drains protruding from my torso; one on each end of my TRAM incision, and one each for my new breasts.

With the dinner tray gone, and night having fallen on the city leaving a low hum of traffic from the streets below, I turned on the TV for the first time since the short stint when mom had wanted to watch something. I didn't want to listen to anything up until this night, and I watched the end of *Survivor*.

Just as the last three contestants took their hike to honor their month-long journey and the people they met along the way, I thought back on who I met that week in the hospital. While I may not have been there for 39 days like those *Survivor* contestants, at times, it felt longer.

Along the way, I was thankful for the incredible surgeons who took my body apart and put it back together. One of those physicians, Dr. Esserman, called me at around 10 p.m. the night before to see how I was doing. She was calling from Washington, D.C., where she was delivering information about her cancer studies in an effort to help more women like me.

I don't know how these doctors maintain their grueling schedules. After my breasts had been removed by Dr. Esserman during a long portion of my operation, Dr. Foster stepped in for his reconstruction task to complete the 10-hour surgery. I am truly amazed and in awe of their achievements and contributions to science and medicine. I was impressed by their intern doctors, nurses and so many others who support what those surgeons do to help women like me.

Aside from that one male nurse who beat the shit out of my tit, the nurses who cared for me that week were incredible. They were caring, warm, interested, empathetic, giving, and the list goes on. Anina, Sara, Deysi and more people. Thank you.

Thank you for holding my hand, looking me straight in the eyes and telling me, all the emotions flowing through my crazy mind were normal. Thank you for reinforcing the message, things would get better. Thank you for your honesty about the parts of recovery that would be difficult to endure. Thank you.

I am thankful for the cards, gifts, visits, calls, e-mails and online support offered by so many friends, relatives and even total strangers. One of our family's closest friends gave me a book called *The Soul Bird*. I'd never heard of it and thought it a sweet little book.

I read it out loud to Mark during his visit, and by the last page, this silly little book brought tears to my eyes. J.K., the message was clear as a bell. Thanks for bringing a soulful and meaningful moment to my day as I looked into the future and saw what the months ahead held in store for me.

After those "survivors" on TV met their final challenge and looked forward to their last night on the island, I, too, looked forward to my last night in the hospital.

My journey wasn't over yet, by any means. It would take 10 to 12 weeks or more of convalescing and healing at home; time enough for my body to resemble something normal and for muscles to find their comfort zones. I would still require the help of others as school ended and we transitioned into a summer schedule. I would still need a lot of my mother's help once Mark had to return to work.

Before slipping into sleep after having taken two Percocets, I thought about how I had taken back some control over my life, my future.

The part of my journey that appeared to be over was CANCER! I felt like a sap because tears began filling my eyes just thinking that I DO NOT HAVE TO THINK ABOUT CANCER EVERY DAY! I had a renewed sense of self and empowerment attached to this control.

I eliminated the high threat of cancer to my ovaries and tubes; I eliminated the high threat of cancer by removing my breasts, thereby lowering my chances of breast cancer to significantly less than that of the average woman (one without the BRCA genetic mutation).

Just as Dr. Esserman informed me the night before, by dropping my chances of breast cancer down to about 2 percent, now my mother has a higher chance of getting breast cancer than I do (and she doesn't even have the BRCA mutation).

So now what? How about something silly...

After my husband's visit and with information offered during a phone call from our home, I realized there had been a lot more going on at home while mommy wasn't around offering a watchful eye.

So here are the top 10 things my children do when mommy is away for a week:

1. Daddy allowed 12-year-old Jesse to drive the car in the parking lot with Sophie in the car. Good thing nothing happened to my children, or the car. "Well, everyone had left, mommy, so nobody saw us," Jesse told me.

2. Daddy allowed 12-year-old Jesse to drive the car in the *synagogue* parking lot with Sophie in the car just to make sure God was watching and can continue reminding me what a shitty parent I am. At least it was on Sunday and not during Shabbat when the rabbi might have seen what my family was doing. I could see him shaking his head as he's done so many times before.

3. Sophie talked daddy into bringing her to Chuck E. Cheese. Okay, that one I don't care about. If he wants to go there, super. I hate going to that rat hole. And for those animal fans out there; no, I have nothing against rats, for shit sake; my blog's profile picture is a photo of one of our sweet little girls (a rat, that is). I just don't think a rat makes for a very good mascot of a restaurant; makes no sense whatsoever.

4. So where were we? Driving at the parking lot, Sophie's restaurant choice and...Sophie talked daddy into a shopping spree at Toys R Us. Doesn't she have enough crap in her room? What will it take to figure that one out? Oh, and by now you may notice a running theme when it comes to my daughter: yes, she is manipulative and convincing. She negotiates everything and has her daddy wrapped around her adorable, little finger. Moving on.

5. Jesse talked daddy into taking him to Target for a new "Ben 10" action figure. Can't let one child get something without being

balanced with the other.

6. Bubby gave the kids ice cream right before dinner. Then, of course, she wonders why they won't eat their dinner. "Well, I didn't know," is her common ditsy response to that one. It's the same tone of voice as when she calls the house in the middle of the week and asks, "So, what are you guys doing today?" Well, mom, Mark's going to work as he does every day. "Oh," she stretches her response with Judy Holliday innocence.

7. Jesse built armor out of cardboard and tinfoil. No, that's okay; it's creative, but then, bubby encouraged Sophie to punch her brother to see how strong his new armor was. Bad bubby! Bad!

8. Bubby asked if she could take the kids swimming after Sophie begged her to go, even though Sophie sounded as if she were getting sick with a cold.

9. Jesse gets daddy to give him a taste of his Wild Turkey bourbon. It's that Southern background. Yup, he's drinkin' and drivin' by the time he's 12. Isn't there some joke in there about how to tell if someone is a redneck?

10. Number 10 never made it on the page. The Percosets kicked in, and I finally passed out for the night.

CHAPTER 18:
RECOVERY BEGINS AT HOME

"Damn it, Jim. I'm beginning to think I can cure a rainy day!"
—Bones, Star Trek 1967 episode Devil in the Dark

Week one: A shower never felt so good

What a difference a shower can make. After shampooing my hair not once, but three times in an attempt to eliminate the crusty crud holding my hair in some demented version of a beehive hairdo from the sixties, that single shower at the hospital felt more spectacular than any shower after returning home from a dusty camping trip.

I could have had a shower the day before, but my plastic surgeon forgot to mention that. But who cares; I finally washed off all the stinky stickiness that had covered my body. I rinsed away the iodine solution that turned my skin orange. I took one more step toward cramming this nightmare behind me.

Sponge baths don't remove much more than a little perspiration, and the liquid soap the hospital adds to the water leaves a horrible odor on your body. Its sickly-sweet fragrance turns malodorous when combined with your body's drug-saturated sweat. It was enough to make your eyes water. I felt sorry for the nurses who had to be around me and the people who chose to visit.

But that was over. It was "going home day" and I couldn't believe I was ready for it. I could barely move only six days earlier, but by Monday I was getting myself to and from the bathroom. I was ready to escape the hospital and return home to my beautiful children, my husband, the privacy of my home, my cushy bed and more hot showers.

It still hurt to raise my arms to shampoo my hair, but my wonderful hubby would continue to help me with that task over the next two weeks. Actually, it was kind of fun taking a shower with Mark; we hadn't done that in ages.

He would get into the shower with me and gently scrub my back and wash my hair. He had installed one of those removable shower heads on the long extension hoses, and then I could sit on a shower chair while he rinsed my hair and body. He would dry my skin and brush my hair. How did I find a man who took such loving care of me when I needed it most? Such a mench!

Before I left the hospital, I was offered one more trip to happy land before heading off in the car and facing scary bumps in the road. Once more, I was loaded full of medicine: some for pain, an antibiotic, one to relax my muscles, another to relieve anxiety, and something else to prevent the queasy feeling caused by the combination of all the meds.

I don't enjoy feeling out of control, and that's exactly how these medicines make you feel; if only I had been more experimental with drugs when I was a teenager, eh? I never had a desire to take drugs like others in high school and college.

It was time to saddle up and face the drive home, but not before I was transformed into the Michelin Man. By the time I was packed into the front passenger seat of our car, plenty of pillows protected me to ensure I couldn't feel the seat belt. Any pressure from the life-saving strap had been absorbed by the many pillows stacked under, around and on me as they served to protect the TRAM incision and my new breasts.

Traveling in a car was comparable to trying to sleep on my side. In fact, I tried unsuccessfully to sleep on my side at home my first night. After 30 minutes of attempting to get comfy, I had to give up. The only way to get comfortable sleeping and sitting was to include a child's pool raft in the equation. The raft offered relief to the damage on my backside and lower back resulting from too much sitting and laying. Setting myself atop the raft, supplemented by numerous pillows, was the only way to find comfortable positions at home.

If you ever have to be in a hospital for more than a night, try to get one of those air mattress beds that continually modify air levels to contribute to your comfort. As I faced my continuing recovery, I was hopeful my sore lower back would correct itself quickly, but it didn't. Sitting in chairs absent extra cushioning was a painful experience.

Week two: Bored batty

After being home from the hospital for a week, I began going out of my mind with boredom.

I know, I know. I was supposed to be taking it easy and recovering. Every time I tried doing anything slightly normal, I ended up hurting myself. There was this one spot in my new left breast, for instance, wherein I'm convinced the surgeons either tied up the parts too tightly, or perhaps they just left something in there. When I raised my arm, outstretched my arm, or lifted anything heavier than a paper cup, a sharp pain in that spot reminded me that I couldn't perform routine movements as I had formerly completed.

Walking was exhausting. I tried to walk through the rooms downstairs, to the bathroom, to the kitchen. When I returned to my chair—my throne, as the kids called it—I would be nearly out of breath and had to take a nap, veg in front of the TV, or surf the internet.

Going down the stairs in our home and getting set up in my throne would only occur after Mark helped me with my morning shower. Mostly, I could give myself a shower by the second week at home, but I still couldn't reach parts of my back or my legs below the knees without some help from Mark. He would even lift the bottle of body wash to squeeze the soap into my shower puff so I wouldn't have to; the actions of lifting the bottle and squeezing out the contents caused pain.

Still, before I could face the task of taking a shower, I would have to pop some pain medicine so my left breast wouldn't tweak with pain when I lifted my arms to wash my hair.

I wrote all these tedious details in my blog. I wanted others who considered choosing a TRAM to have a clearer picture of what to expect.

I was so bored I could scream (if it didn't hurt to scream, that is).

Once I was settled on my throne in the living room each day, I would get on the computer or watch some TV. I found it odd that I could write, but reading put me to sleep. Even the books on my Mp3 player couldn't keep me awake.

Through the hours and hours of boredom, I sat there getting depressed because I wanted my body to recover more quickly. Being on so much medicine didn't help matters and I just wanted to feel healthy and capable again. I wanted to go out and do stuff, but escaping the confines of our home was exhausting. Heading into the city for various post-op appointments were exciting and simultaneously terrifying when I thought about bumps and potholes in the road. Still, most of the time, it was boring, boring, boring. My poor husband; he took two weeks off from work so he could be bored with me.

Undeniably, I was surprised when he was bored enough to trim the bushes in the back yard. Other than mowing the lawn, usually I was the one who did any real gardening in our yard. It was pleasant to have that break. Although, gardening was something I had enjoyed before this surgery took away my core strength necessary to tug on weeds and stretch my arms out over a bush to reach plants farther back.

I thought I might try painting (a canvas), but that hurt, too. Therefore, I was left to write while *Bridezillas* played on TV in the background. I became a total sucker for that trashy show. It drove Mark crazy.

I started watching *Bridezillas* and *Platinum Weddings* to get ideas for Jesse's Bar Mitzvah. Well, maybe from the *Platinum Weddings* show, not so much from *Bridezillas* that served more as a guilty pleasure.

Thank heavens my friend sent me her month-free coupon to Netflix. I had exhausted regular TV shows, and began watching Netflix movies. The fear of mommy's surgery had worn off and everyone was off doing their own thing.

One day, for instance, Mark would be in the kitchen washing a pan, Jesse would be up in his room playing the trumpet and Sophie; I don't know where she was.

The big excitement in my day was getting up out of my throne to take a walk. My temperature would rise some mornings which probably meant I wasn't walking around enough. I would make myself stand into my stylishly hunched-over fashion because I still couldn't stand up straight due to the TRAM slice.

At this point in my recovery at home, I was more concerned about avoiding Lucy, our bitchy cat, who was trying to trip me any chance she got. And then, there was the car issue.

With Mark home after my surgery, he thought he'd get the cars serviced. Naturally, you know how it goes. There's always a part that's missing, or some other delay.

My car, the humongous "I'm embarrassed to be driving this gas guzzler" SUV, is the vehicle we were going to use to drive into San Francisco for one of several post-op appointments. My car has a much softer ride than Mark's smaller hybrid that rattles your body when traveling over a pimple in the road. During that early time in my recovery, I unquestionably required a smooth ride.

Unfortunately, time grew short before we were to leave on our long drive into the city, and panic set in. Panic, because I certainly didn't want to feel every bump in the road in Mark's car; anxiety because his many calls to the car dealership imploring them to complete their task fell on unsympathetic ears.

"Ask if they'll give us a loaner. A big, comfortable car," I begged. He did call them again, and they sent us to the neighboring car rental place. The dealership paid for a small car and Mark upgraded to a sofa on wheels. When he showed up with the cozy Chrysler with cushiony leather seats and shocks that would pacify any ornery senior citizen, I was quite relieved and prepared to face our journey.

On the way into San Francisco, Mark was his usual goofy self to keep me in a merry spirit and my mind off any pain. He would make funny faces every time I attempted to take a photo of us riding in our softened support. Of course, I suppose I kept him chuckling every time I barricaded my body with pillows until I was packed in like a fragile crystal vase being sent off to another country.

"You look great!" That's what was said by everyone at the offices of my surgeons. Nurses, interns and surgeons all came in to see my progress. "You're so ahead of the curve," they said.

"You're kidding?" How can they say that? I can't stand up straight. My belly button is causing all sorts of problems; leaking stuff and looking rather odd. There was pain and....

"Really. You're recovery is going so well." They were all so excited. Watching their unusual display over matters ordinarily repulsive to the general populace—the bruised and scabby scars, the bloody, foul-looking belly button, the black, wiry stitches holding my breasts in place—was like witnessing a slew of entomologists at a bug convention thrilled to see the newest spider species that chews on flesh and shits platinum.

I'm not someone who easily accepts compliments or good news, but I tried believing their cheery outlooks. I couldn't imagine the horrors their other patients experienced during their recoveries if mine was vastly better than most.

While I found it difficult to believe how wonderful they thought I looked, I was happy just to have three of my four JP drains removed. They weren't suctioning out much excess bloody fluid from the areas around my incisions. Having these drains removed is a bizarre procedure.

I have been told by other women, it can be a painful process as these long white tubes are pulled out of your body like some alien tape worm. Still, I had no trouble with mine. It felt more strange than painful, as though someone was tickling your belly on the inside.

Being back at UCSF, it was comforting never having to explain to anyone why I chose this surgery. It was another thing all together at Sophie's school a day later.

It was the evening of open house and Sophie couldn't wait to tell us about all her classroom projects. Also, we would use the event to check out potential teachers for the following school year.

I had been using a cane during short walks when we went to doctor's appointments, and so on, but when I knew I wouldn't be able to sit for a while, Mark would retrieve the wheel chair from the back of the car and use an extra pillow on the seat. I sat in the cushioned wheel chair for her open house so I wouldn't have to suffer through standing for too long, walking too far, or trying to sit my butt down in one of the mini chairs in her classroom.

Suddenly, those friends and acquaintances who didn't know or had forgotten about my surgery were asking me what happened. Others just stared as Mark pushed me about in my wheelchair.

"Oh, I had a big surgery," I'd answer several people.

"I didn't know you were sick," another mom and others said upon seeing me in a wheelchair and finding out I had a mastectomy. Hmm. How do I answer that one?

"No, I wasn't sick. I don't have cancer," I responded.

"Oh," they sounded surprised and looked confused.

Shit! Now I have to explain my situation, because who in their right mind would cut off their tits if they don't have cancer? "Actually, I have a genetic mutation and...," blah, blah, blah. Explain it again to another person whose expression transforms from one of caring and worry to looking as if they feel cheated by stolen sympathy after assuming I was a victim of the "C" word.

I couldn't wait until my body healed enough and I wouldn't have to explain my decision. *Yes, dad, I know. Who cares what anyone else thinks?* It's not that easy. And it doesn't help that I should have to defend my decision at all. I know it's unnecessary to explain, but people want to know; they just don't want to know too much.

Two weeks from the day of my surgery, I found it amazing how the body heals itself; how this machinery of cells and energy combine to create skin that recovers and grows and mends. No, I'm not talking "miracle" shit. Don't expect that from me. And anyway, the body mends; the mind generally takes longer. At any rate, everyone asks, "So, how are you doing?"

Do I tell them the reality? Do I say what I'm really feeling? I figured it probably wasn't best to tell the truth. People don't want that kind of unfiltered information, do they?

If I told them the truth, it would be like the time I went to the synagogue to pick up the kids from Hebrew school when a friend asked, "So, how are you doing?" I paused before answering, assessing what I could say in response. I had known this woman for a while and felt we had developed a reasonably open friendship.

"Well, I've got my period, terrible cramps, a migraine and I feel like shit." Wrong answer.

She just looked up at me with surprise and answered, "More than I needed to know, but I hope you feel better soon."

Perhaps I need to reevaluate my social filters.

So, too much honesty; but fuck it. That was back when I actually got my period; before a doctor told me, they needed to rip out my ovaries and take away any chance of conceiving children in the future. It's not that I wanted more children. Still, it's just not having a choice in the matter that really irks me; there's not even the possibility of having a child because of a happy accident. *Yes, mom. I know I'm repeating myself, but this shit runs through my mind on a regular basis.*

Well, then why did you have your ovaries removed, I can hear the argument. With my odds of getting ovarian cancer, likely you would do the same.

Now, I have too many opportunities for people around me (strangely enough, it's usually my mom, but that's because of how much time we spend together) to see an infant in someone else's stroller before commenting about how maybe I should get pregnant again. My mother doesn't remember saying this, but I know she did. It was difficult to hear. I don't say anything when people make these comments. And then, sometimes, they remember, I can't get pregnant. Not even if I wanted to; I can't because of this blood-thirsty genetic mutation that has left my body ravaged from multiple surgeries.

Okay, too much? Again? Fuck it. If I can't say these things out loud because of societal restrictions, then at least I can spew my emotions and thoughts and fears on these pages. Read the words if you want. Don't if it bothers you. It's everything that's inside me.

I suppose that means (I hope) my written thoughts are like my mother's paintings; her masterful ones that hang in museums. Those are the ones that reveal her darker side; not the commercial crap (no, mom, your painting isn't crap. You know that; it's just what we call the art that sells in touristy stores). If I could write my feelings into a song, I would. Unfortunately, I'm not that clever.

For many years, I wasn't allowed to say anything disturbing to anyone. Wait. I need to clarify that. It wasn't that I couldn't say anything; my family learned quickly, it didn't make sense to tell the truth because people couldn't relate to our experience. It was during the years after Renee was killed.

Yes, I say she was killed because when you're a passenger in a car, and you don't have control over that car when the driver runs it into a massive tree, then it means you are killed; you don't just die from a disease, nor jumping off a bridge for that matter.

For years, people would ask how I was doing after Renee died. It wasn't the right thing to do to tell them the truth. How am I doing? I'm doing shitty. I feel like a huge part of my life has been torn away. It is unfair and ridiculous and cruel. It regularly rips through my mind, heart, stomach, head. It makes me physically ache and ill. I became angry that my childhood was frayed while people asked such an uncomplicated question that should require a complex answer.

Those who asked didn't genuinely want to know the truth because they couldn't, nor were they expected to, do anything to make me feel better. They wanted to hear I was fine, getting along better every day; but only time eases the pain of a death. And time has eased that pain in many ways. Time doesn't remove the pain, it only helps you not think about it too much; time helps you survive absent the person you thought you'd never be able to live without. It was nice of all those faceless people to ask how I was doing after she died, and I apologize if I offered a bitchy response. I'm sorry if I wasn't as polite as I should have been in response to your courteous, obligational question.

Time. Here I am again hoping time is on my side and will heal the physical side of my recent surgeries, as well as the mental aspects of losing parts of who I am.

In keeping with the direct nature of my blog (and personality), I decided to post the "after" photos after having already displayed the "before" photos. Considering I wanted to help other women facing this process, I debated about how much of my body to reveal online. I had watched some YouTube videos of various women showing their post-mastectomy breasts, but I didn't feel comfortable just standing there and taking off my shirt as these women had done. And yet, I wanted women considering a TRAM to have a clearer understanding of what they are getting themselves into.

I decided the only way to exhibit the scars left on my breasts was to show close-up photos of the circular scars that remained; these bruised and swollen lumps which now were absent areolae and nipples. After all, it was just my stomach skin attached to any remaining breast skin to hold it all together.

While I would have never before considered showing my breasts (uncovered) on the internet, after my surgery, these masses of skin attached to my body didn't actually seem like breasts to me; at least, not yet (if ever). They didn't look the same, nor did they feel the same.

A small section of belly is exposed inside the round scar, but the remainder of my heavier belly meat is tucked inside, under the skin to form the breast mounds.

Eventually, when they resemble breasts, they will never lactate, never experience the sensation brought about by a lover's touch. Instead, they will remain numb or no more sensitive than running your fingers across your elbow.

I'm honestly not trying to sound bitchy or angry as my mother says I do. I hope you'll accept my story for what it is: my experience.

So, how was I doing after two weeks?

The reality: I hurt all the time. I was afraid to move my left arm too much because of that extremely painful spot that reminded me of the surgery any time I outstretched or put the slightest weight on that arm; it would even hurt to rub my hands together when washing and drying them (a terrible situation for someone with OCD). My skin was numb and simultaneously extremely sensitive (or it's everything under the skin that screamed with sensitivity and pain, but I just couldn't tell).

I was tired of not being able to stand up straight because of the colossal scar running across my belly that pulled my torso downward toward my legs. I was tired of being out of breath and fatigued when I walked around my house.

I wanted to feel well again and stop taking all the pills. I missed sleeping on my side or wholly reclined. I missed being able to drive. One night I actually had a dream about driving and woke up so happy that I'd been able to drive again. Still, I hated going out in the car; it would be more than a month or more before I stopped traveling in a car with several pillows protecting me from seat belts hurting my chest and stomach wounds; I became terrified of bumps in the road that would jar my body and create pain.

I missed being able to hug my kids or my husband because everyone was afraid they would hurt me. Regardless of Mark saying he was more relaxed being at home, I was worried about my husband's stress level from taking care of me and the kids. And I was terrified about him returning to work and leaving me alone with our children when I was still having trouble getting around.

Okay, enough! Again, you ask, how did I feel?

"Oh, I'm fine. Yup. Getting better every day."

CHAPTER 19:
A TEAR IS ALL IT TOOK

"Come on. Let us take you guys to lunch and get you out of the house," mom told Mark over the phone one morning after I'd been home from the hospital for more than two weeks.

About an hour later, my parents arrived in our area and waited for us at a nearby restaurant for a late lunch.

Sitting in my dad's spare wheel chair, Mark rolled me to a table in the back where my parents were already seated.

"Would you rather take a cruise or go to Hawaii?" asked mom. "Could we take the kids out of school for a week? When is their spring break?"

"April, I think."

"That's too late," mom pondered.

"I thought you were going to Greece in May?" I asked. My mom had recently inherited some money, and it had been burning a hole in her pocket. For years, my sister and I knew we'd never see a dime of our parent's money (if they ever had any) because my mom isn't exactly a miser.

"Well, the plan is...," mom always gets excited when she begins telling about a new adventure.

Their trip to Antarctica the year before had whet their appetite for more travel. That month-long trip included wandering through South America and cruising south over rough seas to complete a journey most people would never consider, especially at the age of 78 like my dad was at the time.

But something was different in her tone. She began detailing what appeared to be a rushed bucket list.

"We're going to start off in England with your sister...."

"You're taking Michelle?" My sister travels better by herself than she does with family. Her hyper and often rude character generally adds stress to family travel. Within two days of leaving, often there's a battle of some sort.

"Yes, she's going to stay with her best friend there for a couple of weeks and show us around. Then, we'll fly on to Greece and take a cruise around the Mediterranean, ending up in Barcelona." Mom and dad wanted to revisit some of the places they had lived when they were first married; when my Air Force dad had been stationed overseas.

"And when are you doing this?" I asked. "In May, right?"

"Well, maybe sooner than that. Maybe we could fly into Florida and meet you guys for the Disney Cruise on the way back!" Mom had wanted to take that cruise since they started offering them.

"Could we go to Disney World? I've never been there. Maybe we could stay at that jungle hotel or the big mountain lodge," I said.

"How soon could we get the kids out of school?" mom pressed for an answer. Sitting around the square table, mom sat to my left, dad was across from me and Mark was to my right.

This was all very exciting to consider, but something was off.

"What's going on? Why the sudden urgency?" I asked her.

Then, I noticed it. Her eyes were welling up with tears. She tried hiding the stress growing in her face. "Mom, what's going on? You're crying. Why are you trying not to cry?" Addressing her tears prompted her to lose control over her emotions.

"Okay. Remember how they thought I was having a heart attack a couple weeks ago?" She'd been leaving one of my dad's many doctor's offices, and during the short walk back to her car, she began having shortness of breath and other heart attack symptoms. She was rushed to the hospital, given six nitroglycerin tablets and kept overnight for observation. Her heart turned out fine.

"Yeah."

"Well, they want to check out my lungs."

Shit! Lungs. Lung cancer? Shit! "What? Why?"

"There might be...," *please don't say the "C" word, please don't say cancer!* "There might be something on my lungs. Maybe polyps." It wasn't polyps, as I found out. She remembered wrong what they told her, or they gave her the wrong description.

"What does that mean? Does that mean cancer? What are they doing? Do you have an appointment for tests?"

My mom tried to remain calm. "It's sometime in late June. They're doing a CT scan."

Remember that horrible night at the hospital when she was angry and picking a fight? Well, here was the reason.

"Late June! If this were me, you would get me into the doctor tomorrow. So why don't they get you in there sooner? Nothing can happen to you, mom." *You're my strength!* "They can't make you wait. That's crap! Is this cancer? What is it?" I started crying thinking about the possibility of my mom going through cancer hell after she's gotten everyone else through all their shit.

She took care of my grandparents until they died, her aunt until she died only a few months before my surgery, my sister's cancer twice, dad's failing health because of his diabetes: heart, strokes, kidneys, increasing blindness, and more. I couldn't fathom the idea of losing my mother to agonizing lung cancer.

At first I thought, this sucks because mom never smoked; a joint or two, but never a ciggy. But then I remembered, I may not have grown up with any smoking in the house, but that's because mom stopped smoking when she got pregnant with me.

She had smoked for many years during the era when doctors would get on TV and say how safe and tasty smoking was. Then, she stopped for good when I showed up around the same time dad got out of the Air Force. Before that time, she describes hanging out with the officers' wives and everyone always had a cup of coffee and a cigarette while all the kids played together.

Dad never smoked. Wait, I take that back. When he was only 12 years old, his mom caught him smoking. Apparently, there were numerous smokers in his family, including his mother, if memory serves. Anyway, she made a deal with her son. She told my dad, if he wouldn't light up another cigarette until he turned 16, she would buy his first pack herself. Dad never smoked again.

"Don't worry. It's probably nothing. A lot of people have these growths, and they just watch them," she said, trying to control her own tears so I would stop crying. "It's not like your cousin. The smaller the dots on the lungs, the worse it is. That's what your cousin Noah says. But it's probably not that. And if it *is* like that, I just want to have fun, and travel and enjoy myself while I can."

"But I thought you said they think it's just these polyps. Can't they get you in any sooner?"

"Don't worry, Joey." I could tell she didn't want to mention any of this to me earlier, or when I was in the hospital. Clearly this had been on her mind, and then it got to be on all our minds until we get any more news.

Thankfully, over the next couple years, whatever was on her lungs went away. One less cancer victim in the family.

CHAPTER 20:
I OWE HOW MUCH?

"Are you ready for this?" asked my husband who was holding a stack of papers after retrieving the day's mail. He hesitantly handed over the pages. It was the hospital's bill for my TRAM surgery.

"Fuck me," I muttered. It was more than $91,000. I felt sick to my stomach.

"You've got to be kidding me," I said as I looked over the pages and pages of itemized costs. The hospital room alone was nearly $5,200 a night. I was there for six nights, thus you do the math.

"You could have stayed at the best hotels with a private nurse and room service for those prices," said mom. Of course, I called her and my dad when we caught our breath after seeing the bill. "For that price, they should have at least given me a fucking bed," mom insisted.

"And this doesn't even include the surgeon's or anesthesiologist's bills," added my husband.

"I want a copy of your bill," said mom.

"What for?" I asked.

"I want to send it to President Obama and tell him how ridiculous our health system is," she said. She and my dad are solid democrats. "So how much is this going to cost you?"

Mark explained the insurance hadn't kicked in yet. Consequently, we would have to wait and see what our final bill would be. "But it will still likely be several thousand dollars," he added.

I thought about what this was going to do to our financial situation and likely how we would have to take out a loan to pay for all this shit plus Jesse's Bar Mitzvah.

But then I said, "You know, this is all because of dad's shitty genes, so I think he should pay for it. Kinda like a wedding of sorts." Everyone laughed. Mark liked that idea. I know, I'm a shitty daughter for throwing guilt on my dad for something out of his control, but it's a crappy situation. Whether or not they like to admit it, everyone tries to place blame on someone or something else. And anyway, I'm Jewish. We do guilt remarkably well.

Oh well, fuck it. What price do you put on life, right? If I have a longer life with my children and husband, it's worth every dime. Especially Dr. Ng who did a superb job and made sure my throat didn't hurt after the surgery. And it was worth getting the epidural of drugs; having it stuck in my spine wasn't exactly fun, but it kept me numb for a few days; therefore, that was worth the price, as well.

Regardless of the bills, my OCD didn't kick in any worse. Prior to the surgery, Mark teased me that I was up to one pack a day (paper towels, not cigarettes). Once I returned home, I got myself down to about five paper towels a day; likely because I remained on my throne too much and I didn't walk as often as I should have.

To that end, Mark came up with a little enticement to get me up off my ass. He led me around the house with a bakery good he held just out of reach. It was a lip-smacking key lime cupcake from the Sift Bakery in Cotati. He turned on the video camera and taped "Cupcake Cam."

After three weeks of healing, here's how my recovery was progressing:

First, some bad news.

I was walking more (in the house), but after two laps through the first-floor rooms, the muscles that carry the blood flow to my new breasts were stretched to the max. It felt as though there were all these bungee cords attached from my waist up to my shoulders that were too short and tugged me downward with each exhausting step. Ten laps through the house; that was about all I could take.

My neck was killing me from sitting up too much throughout the day and night. Mark bought a memory-foam travel neck pillow to help; the kind in a shape of a "U" that wraps around your neck. You may not think so, but sleeping flat at night is just enough time to give your neck a rest from a full day of holding your head upright. I couldn't lie on my side without pain and lying on my back made me feel as if I were going to suffocate.

I was tired of being trapped inside a body that couldn't do normal things. There were too many pills to take every day, every few hours. Acid from my stomach had begun bubbling up into my throat after consuming two different antibiotics, pain pills, anti-inflammatory pills, and more pills.

I longed to have a reduced pain level so I could drive my car again (without the protection of several pillows). I missed driving. I just wanted to stop feeling constant pain for which I had to take pills to dull the discomfort. I hated taking pills because they made me sleep too much. I figured, if I could get off the damn pain medicines, I may be able to drive with my pillows. My teeth began hurting because of all the medicine I was taking.

I was still frightened about facing the first evening alone without someone to help. After those two weeks at home, Mark would return to work. I hated the idea of having my 12-year-old son burdened with doing things I normally did to care for our family.

I began staying up too late because I loathed going to bed. Once I was propped up on all my pillows in bed, I generally sat there in the dark unable to sleep; I couldn't sleep because I was sitting nearly upright.

My spreading, pseudo belly button hole appeared to be drilling deeper and deeper into my stomach. It was bizarre being able to see the meat of my stomach just beyond the top layer of skin.

Okay, enough bitching! Now, the good news.

I began having an easier time doing certain things. I could use my arms a bit more with a little less pain or strain on my new breasts.

I watched some of the video from that first week in the hospital. The nurse who told me several months prior what recovery was going to be like was right; I can't believe I made it through that first horrible week.

I was taking showers by myself, saving one limitation; I was screwed if I dropped something in the shower and nobody was around to pick it up. My method of retrieving something off the floor looks like some spastic character on Monty Python.

Jesse did exceptionally well at his swim meet one of those weekends after returning home from the hospital. In one race, the 200-meter relay, he anchored the race and his outstanding stamina carried him past his competition and brought his team into first place. I know this has nothing to do with my surgery, except I wasn't ready to sit out in the cold for several hours; rather, I opted to stay behind. Mark took videos of all his races, and then I could watch them at home. Oy, my little Michael Phelps!

I'm glad I did the surgery in May and prevented the entire summer from being destroyed for my kids.

CHAPTER 21:
ONE MORE SURPRISE PROCEDURE

The day after Sophie's $1,000 procedure to eliminate cavities in our little girl's mouth, I went to one of my post-op appointments to see Dr. Foster and found out I would have to go under the knife one more time. The surgery was set for the next day when he would fix my new belly button that seemed to be growing wider and deeper, boring a hole into my stomach tissue because it wasn't healing properly.

The skin had begun turning a greyish-green zombie color and oozed with puss. When I nudged the skin aside, I could see down into the red underside of my skin, or fatty tissue, or whatever that was. There was an odd odor, too.

I assume they wanted it fixed quickly because they bumped someone else's surgery to fit me in the following afternoon. I wasn't looking forward to another procedure, but I knew if they took care of it quickly, I could heal, heal, heal and maybe even get in at least one camping trip over the summer.

I didn't even want the damn thing to begin with. In one of my pre-op appointments, I had told Dr. Foster I didn't want a belly button to replace my natural one that would be swallowed up by the TRAM procedure as the skin surrounding it was transformed into my new breasts.

"You're the first person who has ever asked me *not* to give them a new belly button," Dr. Foster repeated with surprise at my post-op.

"Well, see? I told you, it wasn't worth it." I honestly didn't see the point of having it. "Do I really need it for anything medically?"

"Well, no." He said.

Prior to the surgery he had explained, creating a new belly button was a matter of maintaining a normal appearance; bringing balance to my stomach. But who really cares if I have a belly button or not? With my side-to-side scar, it's not like I was going to fashion a bikini any time soon. There was nothing normal about how my TRAM surgery would transform my body.

I had told him, I didn't want the damn thing, but he talked me into it. If it is that big of a deal to him, then I thought, *whatever*. I think he wanted the belly button to satisfy his aesthetic perfectionism more than my vanity. Another victim of OCD?

Then the doctor asked another "typical body appearance" question at this post-op turned pre-op. "I can't remember. Do you want nipples? Because we could do that tomorrow at the same time." This was such a surrealistic conversation.

"Nope." Why would I want permanently-raised nipples? Too many women are self-conscious about such protuberances revealing themselves through a shirt, dress, bra. I suppose I'm no different. So, no, I saw no point in living the rest of my life with knobby nipples placed permanently raised on my new breasts.

"What about areolae? You could have those tattooed on your breasts," he informed me.

"Nah. I'm good." Again, what was the point? I suppose these things—belly button, nipples, areolae—are supposed to make me feel more normal. More like a woman? But very simply, my body is no longer normal. My body has been cut, sliced, sewn, stretched, scraped, poked and prodded. Enough is enough.

Aside from planning the next day's surgery, this appointment was focused on removing the numerous stitches on my breasts and extracting the final of four JP drains. This last drain was attached to my abdomen on the right side. I was exceedingly happy to be rid of this thing dangling from my body.

After several weeks of squeezing out all juicy goodness produced by my healing body and hiding the clear silicon suction bulbs under baggy clothes (so neither other people nor I would have to look at the watery blood) I was glad to be rid of the things.

In preparation of the drain's removal, even though my skin was already pretty numb in my belly region, Dr. Foster further numbed the area with some spray foam stuff. After the foam sat on my skin for a few moments and he clipped the stitching holding the tube to my abdomen, with gloved hands, he grabbed hold of the outer tubing and gently pulled out the surprisingly long (about a foot long, I guess) inner, broad, flattened, white tubing that collected post-surgery fluids and carried it into the drains; the bulbs I emptied two to three times each day after measuring and logging the volume of bloody liquid.

At my prior post-op when he pulled out the other three drains, it didn't hurt or feel like much more than an odd tickle. This time, I felt it more; I experienced some discomfort as the tubing exited my body. It was a strange sensation; it was as though my body had begun growing around the tube and was grabbing hold of the hose after having been inside me for three weeks.

We returned home after the appointment, and I prepared for another surgery the next afternoon. Prior to my surgery, I wasn't supposed to eat or drink anything after midnight. Thinking about the long absence of nourishment left me hungry.

I knew it would be like fasting for Yom Kippur and I'm generally not very successful at that. As luck would have it, I had been eating lighter meals anyway.

But what worried me more was the drug factor. I wasn't allowed to take any pain medication after midnight. I feared how my body would ache by that next afternoon.

Yet again, mom kicked into action and would stay at our house with Jesse and Sophie until we returned from the hospital. Thanks, mom.

I must admit, I can be such a bitch of a daughter when I want to pull mom's leg. She's just so gullible sometimes; or maybe I'm a good actress. In telling her about this new surgery, I began our phone conversation with a bad practical joke.

"Mom, I have to have another surgery tomorrow."

"What? Why?"

"We just left Dr. Foster and he said they have to take my stomach out of my tits and replace it with fat from my buttocks."

I'm such a bitch.

"What!" I love pulling practical jokes on my mom, but this time I knew it would be too cruel to carry on.

"No, mom. Actually, he just wants to fix my belly button." She was relieved, but didn't like the idea of my being knocked out again. She made sure to remind me of the dangers which served as catalyst for my "what if" brain to react with its usual worst-case scenarios; and all because of a fucking belly button!

The next afternoon, Mark drove me back into the city so Dr. Foster could clean out and stitch up my pseudo belly button. Yeah, another scar. Whoopee.

It was 2 p.m. when we arrived for the 4:30 p.m. surgery and already I was famished.

Before Dr. Foster came into the pre-op room, the anesthesiologist entered. It wasn't my hero Dr. Ng.

Panic.

It was a guy with what sounded like a German accent. He kept asking question after question about the same thing, and I started feeling as if I were in an interrogation room instead of heading into a quickie surgery.

I know that sounds ridiculous, but I'm Jewish; I don't respond well to German accents. That wasn't the accent I wanted to hear as I slipped into a deep sleep; I already had enough Morphine nightmares. "You *vill* go to sleep. Shnell, Juden! You take a *deep* breath of zee gas. Go to sleep, Juden!" Can't you just hear it? And before you get your panties in a bind, piss off. My dad's family (and some of mom's) was from Germany…before the war.

I became increasingly insecure and anxious about this quick surgery that was only supposed to take less than an hour to complete. I thought, *great. I've already gone through these two very long and serious surgeries, but it's this ridiculous belly button surgery that's going to kill me.*

After the scary German guy had left the room, I whispered my concerns to Mark.

"Why couldn't it be Dr. Ng? I like him and he makes me feel comfortable."

I desperately wanted my highly skilled hero. I felt it was my own fault for having not asked if he was available for this short surgery. I suppose I didn't think I'd be so lucky to get him a third time since the procedure was last-minute and not as glamorous as my other two surgeries. I imagined this was something one of the other staff anesthesiologists could handle.

This other guy came in twice and continued asking the same questions over and over. Finally, he left. The nurse returned right after he walked out.

"I don't suppose Dr. Ng is on call today?"

"I think he might be leaving soon. Why?" she asked.

I explained about his previous participation on my surgeries and voiced my concern, "I guess I'd just feel more comfortable with him."

The nurse tried to reassure me; whoever served as my anesthesiologist would be just as capable. She left the room.

She must have gone to see if Dr. Ng was still at the hospital because, within minutes, he and his entourage entered the room. A wave of relief washed over me. I smiled broadly with the surprise of receiving a delightful gift. My concerns disappeared. No longer would my husband be required to have my tombstone engraved with the epitaph, "Her belly button did her in."

Shortly thereafter, Dr. Foster arrived before I would be rolled into surgery.

"I have to say it; I told you so," I teased my plastic surgeon.

"Yeah, I know," he said as he leaned down to mark his territory writing his initials, "RF," on my belly.

The surgery was uneventful. I remember breathing in through the mask and falling asleep before waking up and being rolled into the quiet recovery room.

I recuperated rather quickly from any anesthesia, faster than the last time I had to get some teeth filled at the dentist. In no time, I was sitting up and eating graham crackers and drinking from small hospital containers of apple juice. The simple fare tasted scrumptious in my growling belly.

I wanted to get out of the hospital. Just after 6 p.m., the nurse finally approved my release, and I didn't waste any time getting ready. I was rolled down to our car before we left for home, but while heading north, we stopped to have dinner at one of my family's favorite haunts: Marin Joe's.

I've been going there since I was a kid, just as my mom had gone to the Joe's in the Marina (in San Francisco) since she was a child. Marin Joe's is always crowded from the moment they open their doors. Lucky for us, we were able to snag a booth in the side room near the piano bar.

Mark and I sat at the corner table. Two youngish couples sat at the booth to my right. The women fashioned standard Marin hardware: $2,000 purses. And carrying on about their Porsches, the men said they can't drive on Highway 5 from Los Angeles without speeding at 105 mph; their infractions get them stopped by police at least once per month.

One woman said she keeps a photo of a police captain friend in her wallet. When she's pulled over (also for regularly speeding), the officer notices the photo and asks who it is. She tells them, "He's my brother," and she gets out of any tickets.

At the table across from us, three alter kakers (Yiddish for old geezers) sat enjoying a few drinks and plenty of Joe's delicious sour dough French bread. One of the men kept sweeping the bread crumbs off the table with his hand and dumping the morsels into his dinner: liver and onions. Yuck! Growing up in the Bronx during the Depression, my dad would tell how eating liver and onions was a treat and became his favorite dish; other cuts of meat were too expensive. Sitting at this table, I just hoped I wouldn't smell the liver.

One of the man's companions ordered rabbit. I only know that because, throughout their meal, one of the chefs made several visits to their table to schmooze about gambling. The chef joshed about about how the other two men's meals were taking longer to arrive because they were waiting for the rabbit to cook.

Watching their interaction with the chef who was doting on the old men was like stepping back in time to watch my grandfather at a San Rafael Italian restaurant owned by one of his childhood friends.

My grandpa was a charismatic, gregarious sort of fellow who moved north from Los Angeles to San Francisco when he was a child. The day he and his family arrived at the train station in San Francisco, his father left the station to find lodging for the night. My grandpa, who was only about 5 years old at the time, was left there with his mother and 8-year-old sister, Ann. Unfortunately, while she was playing at the station, grandpa's sister ended up breaking her arm. Great-grandma took Auntie Ann to the hospital with my grandpa.

But when great-grandma returned to the station, great-grandpa was nowhere to be found. Moreover, she only spoke Yiddish and wouldn't ask the police for help because she considered the police to be like the Cossacks in the old country. Jews never went to "the authorities" for help because assistance was the opposite of what they would receive. And with that, my great-grandmother became a single parent.

The San Francisco train station was located near the Barbary Coast where it wasn't uncommon for people to be shanghaied and sent to work on merchant ships leaving San Francisco. Knowing how much great-grandpa loved his wife and children, our family was convinced he had been shanghaied or killed. Grandpa never learned what happened to his father, and it remained the family mystery.

Eventually, great-grandma and her children settled north of San Francisco in Marin County; they lived in San Rafael located in Central Marin.

As a single parent, great-grandma was always working to sustain her family. During those difficult years, grandpa had befriended his life-long best friend, Leo. Leo was one of a dozen children in an Italian Catholic family. Soon enough, grandpa spent more time at Leo's house than his own. As he put it, in Leo's house, one more mouth to feed wasn't going to make a difference. Grandpa called Leo's mother "mama" and eventually moved in for a few years because great-grandma couldn't support her family when she became ill. She was doing the best she could manage under terribly difficult circumstances at a time when there were no social services to help.

It was Leo's family and his friendly wife who owned an Italian restaurant in San Rafael. The restaurant's unusual sign displayed the name clearly marked on a boat propped high up on a post; it could be easily seen from the east side of Highway 101.

Periodically, our family would dine there because grandpa loved Leo's family's Cioppino recipe. And every time we went, Leo would linger at our table, schmoozing with grandpa and offering delectable cuisine for his best friend's family.

Therefore, after grandpa was raised on Italian food, it's no wonder why to this day, my favorite food is Italian. Just as I was raised on a lot of delicious Italian meals, so was my mom when she was a child living in the predominantly Italian Catholic Marina neighborhood of San Francisco.

I know it's not beneficial to find comfort in food, but feeling a little normal by going to Joe's precisely was what I needed that evening after my navel was closed to became a new BRCA battle wound.

Chapter 22:
One month after my TRAM

When the first month of recovery from my TRAM surgery came to an end, it was hard to believe so much time had passed. Again, that nurse was right. I would look back on those early days after the surgery with amazement I managed to survive.

By the end of the first month, I was walking around my house, but still, the longer I walked, the more hunched over I became as though someone had been pulling me downward. Regardless, it was good to be able to walk around more.

What I truly missed, aside from not feeling pain all the time, was being able to walk without effort. I kept having dreams about mundane tasks.

I would dream about taking a brisk hike and how delightful it felt to do so. I would dream about picking up objects that weigh more than a glass of water and not feeling like I just pulled my stomach muscles out of whack. I would dream about reaching for objects on a top shelf in the kitchen cabinets. In the dream, I could reach items easily absent pain or feeling as though I was ripping something out of the side of my body with a tugging and tearing sensation inside my breast.

Each night, I thought about what I would be able to do the next day. I thought using imagery would help me achieve these goals, but mostly those images resulted in wishful thinking as I set myself up for failure.

Invariably, I would end up sitting on my living room throne, holding off from taking pain killers for as long as I could stand it before succumbing; I'd take a pill and feel drowsy and watch more movies.

Most of the time, any attempt at creative writing was useless; my senses were dulled by drugs and more drugs. I didn't have the energy to finish writing any story and continually doubted my writer's voice would reach anyone and impact someone's mind, spirit. I assumed whatever I was writing was boring crap because I wasn't doing anything interesting. I continued chronicling my recovery and BRCA experience, but I wasn't sure if anyone was reading my blog.

That is until people began commenting on my story. At first, people (mostly women) commented on how brave I was to go through this TRAM process, especially not having cancer. When I started blogging about my journey, I decided I would be honest and tell all the details of this barbaric surgery. It turns out, that is what the readers enjoyed and respected; they were hungry for more information.

The women who had breast cancer and the women who were BRCA positive; they wanted all the horrific details the physicians wouldn't reveal. These readers were supportive of my proactive journey. Some suggested the surgeons read my stories to secure better understand how to help others facing this process.

In response to one comment about the lack of information provided by the medical field, I responded by saying, "I agree with you that the surgeons never tell about those types of things that can go wrong. They might skim the surface, but I imagine women wouldn't go through with it if they really knew what to expect. The "docs" on *Grey's Anatomy* give out more pre-surgery details than the real surgeons do."

My sister, as well, had experienced this frustrating lack of information, I wrote to a reader. "Before the hospital began the bone marrow transplant process on Michelle the first time she had breast cancer, all they said was, this is going to hurt."

I shouldn't admit this, but I'm glad I wasn't in her room that day. I couldn't be there because I was sick with a cold; therefore, I was told to stay away. Mom told me how she watched Michelle transition from calmly laying in her bed, to screaming and crying in agony as though she was being burned from the inside out.

In the several days leading up to Michelle's bone marrow transplant, mom described the scene with the numerous bags hanging by my sister's bed. She was being pumped full of chemotherapy.

"They gave her so much chemo, she was on the verge of

death," said mom.

The chemicals would kill off the white blood cells and leave her with neutropenia: her body couldn't fight off any infection (including my cold, at the time). Any such infection could kill her.

Back then, the chemo they offered my sister made her terribly ill and the anti-nausea drugs didn't prevent the repetitive vomiting that resulted in canker sores lining her throat; sores that left her in agony every time she puked up the acidic juices from her stomach. That first week in the hospital, mom said all Michelle did was cycle through sleeping and vomiting.

"When she was awake, she was in agony. There was absolutely nothing I could do," mom said. "You feel helpless."

Mom remembered Dr. Gloom visiting during that awful first week in the bone marrow transplant ward and telling Michelle, if you think this is bad, don't worry; it's going to get worse. Dr. Gloom or Dr. Doom: those were our names for Michelle's oncologist. His personality was absent any warm and fuzzy bedside manner, but he got the job done.

One afternoon, when watching her daughter suffering became too much, mom went out into the hall and sat on the floor outside Michelle's room. Next to her sat another mother on the hall floor outside her son's room. He was in his 20s.

The two mothers spoke about their helplessness. The other mother told my mom how there was nothing more to be done to help her son. He cried out in agony, but nothing could diminish his pain. He died that same night.

"It's like you're out in the ocean and you see this enormous wave coming at you, and you know there's no escape," mom said.

Walking the halls during those weeks in the hospital was a disheartening experience for my mother. Several other bone marrow patients died during those weeks; she would overhear mothers calling their family to tell about another heartbreaking death.

As well, she would have to dodge items patients threw at the nurses, or out into the hall. One patient would throw his bed pan or dishes and scream how he wanted to end the torment and the few days remaining of his life.

Being an artist, mom transformed her feelings and impressions into drawings. Eventually, two of her sketches, complimented by Michelle's descriptions written on those works, would be included in the book *Art.Rage.Us: Art and Writing by Women with Breast*

Cancer (Chronicle Books, 1998).

After six days of killing off her malfunctioning bone marrow and blood cells, it came time to give her the life-saving blood stem cells. Again, I'm not an expert, but in lay terms, it is the bone marrow (a spongy material found inside some bones) that produces infection-fighting blood cells. This process kills off the faulty bone marrow before healthy stem cells are put into the blood stream. If the process works correctly, the transplanted cells begin producing healthy cells; otherwise, she would have died.

Just as my sister's chemo experience dramatically improved with her second breast cancer, I've been told the current bone marrow transplant technique isn't the painful process it had been for her at the end of 1994. Now, bone marrow recipients receive the stem cells via an IV drip over the course of several hours. It wasn't like that for my sister.

When the day arrived that Dr. Gloom would inject the stem cells into Michelle, he used massive syringes filled with something that looked like watery tomato soup. Dr. Gloom plunged the life-saving juice into my sister's chest IV line using needles mom compared to something out of a horror movie.

Almost immediately, Michelle experienced pain, cramping, nausea. My sister can't talk about that time without feeling nauseated. Yet, she did tell me, after the first injection, "Every orifice wanted to expel at the same time." There was convulsive vomiting, uncontrollable urination, explosive diarrhea, stabbing gas pains.

She remained in agony as cold, calm Dr. Gloom said, "Just a little more." He plunged the contents of the second syringe into my sister. With that, he said, "Okay. That's it," and left.

That day, there had been a photographer from a local TV news station recording the process for a story. News photographers see a lot of nasty shit in this world; but on that day, he had to leave the room. My sister's suffering had been too much to watch.

"After the transplant, we waited to see if the damn cells would come back," said mom. That waiting game took more weeks in the hospital.

As frustrating as my sister can be at times, she turned out to be a model patient. The nurses complimented her effort, cooperation and compliance during that month.

"They liked Michelle. Before she left for home, they had

stopped by her room and congratulated her," mom said.

The day Michelle returned home, she was so weak she had to be carried into the house. Still, she wasn't going to give up her fight.

The next morning, my parents were surprised when said she wanted to go to the park to take a walk. They took her to Pioneer Park in Novato where there were vast lawns and old trees lining the paths of this popular picnic and summer "outdoor movie" destination.

Michelle took two steps forward, and that was all she could manage. Regardless, they returned every day, and she would walk a little farther. A month later, she was walking around the park and completing the circular path.

"Dad and I gained enormous respect for her strength. By God, she wasn't going to let cancer beat her," mom said.

Later, my sister told me, had she known how truly miserable the process was going to be to complete this bone marrow transplant, she wouldn't have gone through it. Okay, well, I guess that's why they don't tell anyone. If you are about to have a bone marrow transplant, please ignore this; I wouldn't want someone to pass up a life-saving procedure because of my sister's hindsight. I truly hope the process indeed has improved to remove the intense pain she and others experienced years ago. But she's alive today, years later. Therefore, our family must say it was worth the pain. Of course, that's easier for me to say than my sister.

I've always considered Michelle to have a much higher tolerance for pain than I do. If the government wants to torture someone, it shouldn't waste its time with waterboarding. That's child's play in comparison to what my sister endured with her cancer treatments, or my TRAM, for that matter. Put people through TRAMs, breast cancer treatments, bone marrow transplants. I'd rather go through one of my very long, hard labors than experience another TRAM. At least the pain from childbirth goes away, and you're left with a beautiful little prize.

On one of my blogs, a woman said she considered me courageous and said, "A brave lady like you will be an inspiration to many more."

I told my family about these comments and how it made me feel really good knowing I was having an impact on the world. Even if what I wrote provided a small impression, my story began making a difference. Women were hopeful.

I was getting contacted by women (and still do regularly, a few years later). Some women would want to chat on the phone and I began speaking to women from all over America, Canada and beyond our shores.

Some women who thought they wanted a TRAM would realize, ultimately, it wasn't the best choice for them. And for others, knowing what to expect helped them prepare for their own TRAMs.

"I've read all of your posts and watched your videos, and I can't begin to tell you how informative they have been for me," wrote Tonia. "Nobody wants to tell you the 'bad' stuff. They want to say that you will be sore for a month or so, but that it will get better. I want to *know* what to expect so then I don't freak out about something I shouldn't worry about."

There were many messages like this. Some women posted public comments and others sent private e-mails. What was so frightening about all this was the number of women facing this process. And no matter how much support one gets from family and friends, their solitude and terror had been revealed in their sorrowful stories.

As word spread to other women facing this TRAM procedure, the comments transformed again. Women began telling their own TRAM stories and how they survived. They began helping each other and supporting one another. These brave women were empowering each other as we collectively survived this mastectomy torture chamber.

It was these messages and the growing conversation that occupied my mind with a message of hope during those tedious hours of boredom during my recovery.

There were times when I thought I was going bonkers as my body healed and my mind raced to catch up with all the changes that were laying the foundation to impact the rest of my life. Aside from the large supply of pain medicine, there were other drugs that were supposed to help me pull through this trying time and keep me from going insane.

Still, all this boredom and drugs sent me into a minor depression. I say "minor" because, no, I wasn't going to kill myself. I was just bored and ready for my body to be healthy.

I hate sitting still and doing nothing. I'm one of those typical Americans who don't know how to relax without accomplishing or creating something. I feel guilty if I just sit around and watch TV. I might be painting a picture, crafting, sewing, writing, or designing something on my computer. Sitting and doing nothing; most certainly, that was not for me.

"Just relax and take it easy. Allow your body to heal." That's what everyone said I needed to do, and they were right. I just didn't have to like it.

With one month having already passed, I would be closer to feeling like myself again (I hoped). In another month, I would be driving my children to all their activities. Normally, I considered that more of a burdensome chore, but now I invited this task I previously had taken for granted. And as my health improved, camping became an option. I could enjoy some summer fun with my family.

Until that time arrived, I would continue thinking about all the things I wanted to finish while I was stuck in the house, sitting on my throne. The belly button surgery added a little more time to my recovery, but I was happy to be down to one bandage; that allowed me to take showers more easily.

And one more shower update. Unlike a couple weeks prior, by this time if I dropped something, I was able to lean down to pick up items off the floor if I were particularly careful. It hurt to do so, but I was able to stretch a little more.

I would also continue caring for the dressing on my non-belly button. The dressing that was supposed to cover my closed pseudo belly button for the entire two weeks prior to my next appointment began looking rather gross; the dressing had become bloody and soggy. We called the doctor, and they said to change the waterproof dressing.

That gave me and Mark a chance to check out my non-belly button; it looked pretty cool. It wasn't gross and covered in green goo as we were afraid it might be. Instead, it was dry and on the road to recovery. With these additional 12 stitches, I looked like Frankenstein with all my scars. Scars which my sister says don't even come close to all the scars she has; now that's a bizarre form of sibling rivalry.

Those stitches were removed two weeks after the surgery. The way it was healing, my belly button began to look like an "outie". Eventually, the scar that tugged on the skin would flatten out before becoming an ever so slightly "innie."

I imagine there will come a day when my son returns home with his friends who want to see my non-belly button. Yippee, I'll become a sideshow freak. Can you imagine the look on the coroner's face when they take a look at my body on the slab some day? That is, many, many years from now, I hope, because I'd hate to go through all this shit just to get run down by a bus or something.

My family knew my recovery was going to be a long process, but I was surprised by my dad's reaction to a question he asked. One afternoon, my parents arrived to help with a driving task for the kids. My dad slept in a chair most of the visit as was common those days. When he awakened, he asked how I felt.

"There's constant pain all the time. It's getting better, but it's always there," I told him.

"Joey, I've been in pain the past 30 years, but you don't hear *me* complaining about it," he responded.

Yes, dad, I know you don't complain about it, but you did ask how I felt, and I did have a surgery that makes me feel like crap. If you don't want to know, don't ask. I chalked up his comment to being old and having lost his mind after several strokes.

By this time in my recovery, I still wasn't getting out of the house too much, although Mark tried to bring me out for lunch now and again. More often than I should have, I turned down these offers to escape the confines of our home; going out would tire me for the remainder of the day. I welcomed a few short visits from people, but even those social calls were exhausting.

Making matters more complicated, you know how when you lose a part of your body, it is said you may feel phantom parts? That's sort of how it felt on my new right breast. I don't know if it was because of the scabs that grew over the scar, but there was this itch that wouldn't go away.

The surface of my skin was numb, while the nerve endings—or whatever was underneath—were screaming with sensitivity. And then there was this feeling my nipple had an itch. I'm not trying to be crude or anything, but I felt as if I needed to pinch it to eliminate this constant, nagging sensation. But I had no nipple to pinch, grab or scratch. I thought I would go mad. It was like having "restless leg syndrome" in my tit. Aaaagh!

Perhaps it was because the stitches were removed from my breasts, but these new mounds would remain extra sensitive and sore for a couple of weeks.

CHAPTER 23:
GOD'S CRUEL SENSE OF HUMOR

Ladies, have you ever walked into a public bathroom stall, looked in the toilet and, "Eew!" Someone has left a wad of bloody tissue in the bowl. Sure, you could just flush and continue with your business, but when there are more empty stalls, your first reaction is to back away and move on to the next.

That's what happened to me at Macy's one day during the eighth week after my TRAM. With extra cushioning of pillows protecting my belly and breasts, I started driving again about six weeks after my big surgery. My unusual padding attracted a few double-takes from people in other vehicles I passed along my routes.

After I had started driving again, I did what I could to prevent injury. That included changing how I turned the car. Rotating the steering wheel to turn my heavy car would put uncomfortable strain on my stomach muscles, but I figured out a push-pull system. I would keep my hands on the sides of the wheel to avoid my former cross-over style requiring those long stretches of my arms over the top of the wheel; stretching that way would tug on the muscles resulting in what felt like a pulled muscle that would take several hours or a day to heal.

I made the 15-minute drive north to Macy's in Santa Rosa. I was on a mission to find some cute tank tops, and perhaps a pair of pants since all my clothes had dropped two sizes since my surgery (yippee!). Why specifically tank tops? First, a little background story.

When I was a teenager, I remember when my mom suddenly began wearing tank tops all the time. Summer, winter, the season didn't matter; she wore mostly light, airy tops.

After having my ovaries removed, and I experienced the forced onset of menopause, I understand mom's clothing choices. When your face begins flushing and your body feels like you just stepped into a 200-degree sauna, you want to be wearing these light tops so you can cool down quickly. Then, when your hot flash ends, you can return to a freezing state. Hot, cold, hot, cold; no wonder women go bonkers during menopause.

Anyway, after my husband convinced me to go along with him and our son to eat Chinese food for lunch (I'm the only Jew who hates Chinese food), my stomach was churning by the time I arrived at my favorite clothing section at Macy's.

"Can you hold this for me for a few minutes," I asked the woman working the checkout counter and hung a skirt on the rack. I raced away from her station and toward the escalator heading up to the top floor where the restrooms were located.

I walked in, peered inside the stall, and there it was. A bloody wad of toilet paper in the bowl.

Eew. Glad that's one thing I don't have to deal with anymore, I thought before moving on to the next stall. Thanks to the greasy Chinese food, I barely made it onto the toilet after fumbling with the thin seat covers that kept ripping. This is where God's cruel joke took over.

That same afternoon, after a full schedule of driving my children back and forth from music lessons, swim team and Sophie's summer acting camp, I was bushed. Generally on those driving days, I would need to collapse on my reclining chair when we returned home. We almost went to the store to buy something for dinner, but the thought of walking around the grocery store for various meal supplies sounded like a terrible idea that would send me over the edge of fatigue.

"Would you rather have roasted chicken at home, or go out for dinner?" It's not difficult to figure out which option the kids chose. By the time we reached the restaurant, I had to go to the bathroom again. I raced back to the restroom. Sophie accompanied me so she could wash her hands while I sat on the toilet.

"Ouch!" I was crying out as quietly as I could manage.

"What's wrong, mommy?" Sophie asked. Ever since the surgery, my children's concern-o-meter was more alert than ever.

"I don't know," I tried to say calmly. I honestly *didn't* know. I just knew I was suddenly experiencing intense pain when I made a pish (Yiddish for urinating). Sorry to be crude, but it felt like I'd just been fucked exceedingly hard or someone with sharp nails was grabbing hold of my vagina and ripping it away.

But then, it got worse. I wiped away any remaining moisture. There was blood on the wad of toilet paper. "What the fuck?" Don't worry; I don't think Sophie heard me. Anyway, my kids know mommy has a cussing problem.

I can't have my period. I have no ovaries. My mind raced with confusion. *Maybe I hurt myself when I made that turn in the car.* On the way to the restaurant, I had to pull the car through a tight turn and thought the tugging might have pulled a muscle or some stitches loose or something. *No, it can't be that; everything is healing. Hasn't it been too long? I'm not supposed to lift; maybe I caused a hernia or something. They warned me about that.*

And then the thoughts got worse. Maybe it's something else entirely. Spotting, pain…*Oh, shit. Uterine cancer! After all the shit I've been through; and this is what you're going to throw at me? Uterine cancer? You're actually going to brew up a cancer in my genetically fucked-up body to strike the piece of flesh the doctors left inside me? You sick, sadistic, son-of-a-bitch bastard!* (Yes, rabbi, I know I'm a shitty Jew to consider God has nothing better to do than fuck around with my life.)

I didn't want to seem upset around the kids, but they could tell something was wrong. *What do I do? What do I do?* It was already 5:30 p.m. and the doctors' offices were closed. But who would I call anyhow? The plastic surgeon who did the TRAM Flap surgery? The oncology gynecologist who took out my ovaries? My regular Ob/Gyn closer to home?

I went outside and called my mom.

"What's wrong, Joey," mom answered. I explained about the "sharp-nailed vagina grabber" pain and told her about the blood. I tried to hold back tears.

"You need to call your doctor *now*," she said. Which one? "Call the one who took your ovaries. Do it now, Joey." I called the answering service. That wasn't any help. There wasn't much they could do.

"Contact your regular gynecologist tomorrow, or if it gets worse, go to the emergency room tonight," said one of my surgeon's partners who had been on call. Before she gave me that answer, I had compared the pain to one resulting from rough sex, but before I could say more she jumped in. "Oh, did you have sex last night? Because that could be what's causing this and...."

"No, I didn't have sex. It just feels really sore as though...," why was I explaining this? Who in their right mind would feel well enough to have sexual intercourse so soon after having a TRAM Flap slice across their belly? (If you read this and you did, I can't imagine how it felt. Perhaps it would be like how it's frightening to have sex too soon after giving birth.)

I figured, *okay, I can deal with this for a night and call my local Ob/Gyn tomorrow.* The sharp-nailed vagina-grabber bitch rejected that plan.

By the time the kids were getting ready for bed, the pain had become worse. And by 10:30 p.m., peeing was excruciating and there was a growing amount of blood left in the toilet bowl after each agonizing release of urine.

I called Dr. Foster's office and spoke through tears with the doctor on call. He said this likely wasn't associated with my surgery, but if it gets worse I should go to the ER. Once again, I called my mom.

"I'm coming up to bring you to the hospital," she insisted. I couldn't stop crying from the pain and didn't think it would be smart to drive myself up to the hospital with the kids. Mark was still at work in the city and mom could reach me faster. The pain was so severe, I nearly called an ambulance. "Dad will watch the kids, and I'll take you to the emergency room."

A half hour later, dad was at my door; mom had the car running outside. Another 20-minute drive and we arrived at the emergency room in Santa Rosa.

The longer we waited, the more my mom would beg them to bring me back into the exam room because of my agony; she kept telling them about my surgery and how she was worried something had gone wrong. It took more than an hour to see a doctor. By then, when they asked me to provide a urine sample, I was terrified of sitting on the toilet and completing the task.

While walking hunched over toward the bathroom, I held my stomach with one hand and a specimen cup in the other. My hands were shaking when I grabbed for a tissue seat cover. The first flimsy sheet ripped as I pulled it out of the dispenser hanging on the wall. I managed to pull out another seat cover and place it on the toilet before sitting down.

I held the urine cup under me. I gritted my teeth and panted in fear of the excruciating pain that would shoot up from my crotch when the urine began to flow. But worse, when the stream dwindled, the discomfort intensified; I moaned and cried as the bright pink, bloody urine filled the cup.

Before we went to the emergency room that evening, I'd already taken two Aleve, an Ativan and a Percocet, but nothing was helping. Once inside the exam area, an IV was placed in my arm; I was given Morphine to help alleviate the suffering. They conducted a CT Scan to make sure I hadn't ripped anything from the surgery. They checked for any post-op infection (unlikely because it had been nearly two months since the TRAM).

After Mark had arrived at the hospital, mom left at about 3 a.m., only after she knew I was safe and the doctor diagnosed the source of the pain. Mom returned to our house to get some sleep. Mark and I didn't leave the hospital until 5:30 a.m. when the skies were just starting to glow with morning's dim light. Being up so early felt as though we should be on our way to the airport; we should have been catching an airplane to some tropical, fun destination; not returning from the hospital.

Mark took the day off from work to care for me and the kids. He managed to get up early to get Sophie to her acting camp. I slept most of the day away.

So what was all the fuss about? If you haven't figured it out yet, it was a urinary tract infection. I'd had bladder infections while I was pregnant with my son when I didn't drink enough water, but I'd never felt anything like this and certainly nothing that struck with such swift intensity.

Regardless of my doom and gloom thoughts, it was not uterine cancer, thankfully; just a bitch of an UTI with an exorbitant bill attached.

Aside from that infection, two months after the TRAM I was still experiencing a lot of sharp aches in my chest and stomach. The muscles were still pretty tight and hurt most by the evening. I cut down my pain meds to Aleve during the day, and a half (or a quarter) of a Percocet along with an Ativan at night.

Also, starting at about seven weeks after the surgery, I began noticing a different, slightly painful sensation; I would feel tiny, stinging sensations shooting through my chest and sometimes in my abdominal region.

It felt like the time I was snorkeling with my sister in the ocean and we accidentally swam through a swarm of baby jellyfish. We both received several tiny stings that warm afternoon in the Caribbean.

I asked my plastic surgeon about the stinging at a post-op appointment. He said this was a healthy sign that my nerve endings were healing; I might get some feeling back in my breasts and the other areas that feel numb on the skin surface.

I did start to feel a little more sensitivity in my new breasts, but when I ran my hand along the skin of my stomach, it still felt numb to the touch. It felt as if I had been given a bunch of shots of Novocain at the dentist; it was kind of like when you can't feel your lips when you bite down on them.

I wasn't using a cane so much during these days. I tried to walk more and more. It was around this time when I began using my Wii Fit, doing about five to 10 minutes of aerobic step before adding another 10 minutes of less-than-brisk walking on our treadmill. Those 20 minutes of exercise were about all I could manage before the muscles from my stomach leading up to my chest began tugging tighter and tighter.

This struggle to be active was a difficult change considering my vigorous hour-long workout prior to the surgery. I was determined to build my time back up to that amount. It would be a slow process.

Because I still grew tired by the afternoon, Jesse was a terrific helper. He would make dinner for me and Sophie when Mark wasn't home. We had a lot of take-out or easy cooking, quick meals.

My mom may have been a horrible cook when we were kids, but she rarely used canned or prepackaged foods. Just like many women in our family, I'm no master chef, either. When most of my friends in the neighborhood would dine on canned fruits and vegies, mom rarely purchased anything but fresh foods.

Therefore, easing up on that custom was difficult. While I didn't care for frozen, pre-packaged foods, having them in the house made it easier on my children; especially my young son who took on extra responsibility of making many meals for us during the week while Mark at work. I felt badly that we pushed him into this position, but I suppose that's just what families do when someone needs help.

I tried the best I could to return to some previously normal activities. I quickly realized there were some undertakings that would never return; gardening, for instance.

Before the surgery, I loved working in my garden for hours on end. As I healed, I tried doing some light gardening, but I was a shmuck and did too much. Mark would get upset with me for straining my body, leaving me extremely sore and suffering by the evening.

Mowing the lawn and using the weed whacker was the extent of Mark's gardening participation, but we developed a new system to care for the yard. I would sit in a chair in the garden and tell Mark what I wanted trimmed back. This sounded fun at first as a way to boss around my husband, but I used to find gardening quite rewarding and missed the work. Bending over a few times to trim this branch or that bush was all I could do before the muscles begin aching and tugging.

On the surface of my body, by mid-July, I was two small scabs away from the skin healing on my new breasts which were softening up. I still had some nasty red scars, but I was hopeful they would fade in time.

Twice a day, I began using concentrated lotion (Neutrogena Hand Cream) on the scars, working it into the gnarly lines to soften them up. I had looked into some of those creams that are said to be beneficial for scars, but after speaking with my doctors and the pharmacist, they didn't seem terribly impressed by their results. Furthermore, they tended to be much more costly.

I also began going to physical therapy. Twice per week, a woman would massage my new boobs to soften the stomach flesh that formed my breasts. Also, she had to tenderize the solid formation on the bottom-right side of my right breast.

Having someone clinically massage your breasts is an unusual experience. Originally, I was supposed to see a physical therapist up in Santa Rosa; a woman who specialized in working with women who have had mastectomies and related surgeries. Unfortunately, when I called to make an appointment, they said she was taking some time off and wouldn't be available for appointments for a while.

"I don't know if you'd be interested in this, but there's another guy here who does the same work," said the receptionist. I surely didn't want some strange guy massaging my boobs; fake or not. That was too creepy to consider.

"Do you know when she will be returning?"

"Well, we're not really sure," added the woman. "She just found out she has breast cancer and she needs time off for that."

How ironic is that?

I didn't want to drive into the city every other day. Therefore, I returned to a physical therapist nearby who had worked on other parts of my body over the years.

Regardless of the person conducting the body work, it isn't a comfortable situation to have someone massaging and working on your tits. The skin was numb to the touch, but still, it was an odd scene laying there with my shirt off and someone's hand on my breast. It was enough of a stressful situation to trigger menopausal hot flashes which meant my body would turn bright red and perspire. But I suppose this was much easier to go through with a woman rather than a man.

In any case, her methods did help to loosen up the breasts' heavy stomach meat; yes, the stomach fat transferred into the breasts feels much heavier than natural breast material and acts like insulation allowing the heat to linger after a hot flash dissipates. The price of this body work was that it awakened my breasts and increased circulation; it created the feeling of an itch that can't be relieved as you claw at your numb skin.

Both my breasts seemed a bit boxy, but that right breast was a bit larger and those hard lumps stuck out to the side enough to make it uncomfortable against my arm. I often wondered if my surgeon had allowed one of his interns to practice their surgical skills thereby creating that squared tit.

Dr. Foster suggested a quick corrective surgery to provide more symmetry, but I thought I'd wait and see how everything finally healed before jumping into another operation.

I wanted to reinforce my choice not to move forward with another surgery, but I also wanted to make sure I wasn't crazy to wait and miss this opportunity. Concurrently, some of my friends were curious to see how everything turned out. Therefore, this became a good time to reveal my new body to get their opinions on whether or not I should opt for additional corrective surgeries.

I was getting used to the new look of my body, but my friends didn't know what to expect; they weren't prepared for what they saw.

During their visits to my home, when they were ready to look at my new breasts, we went upstairs and away from the living room windows.

"Okay, here are the new girls," I would say and lift up my shirt.

Right away, I'd notice a twinge of shock in their expression. Most did their best to hide any horror at the sight of all my scars. Some of my cousins acted on revealing their feelings.

"Oh my God," said one cousin who was mesmerized by the scars.

"Well, they're still healing," I would defend.

Then, their attitude would change as they recalled why I had taken such extreme measures. They would remind me how important it was that I had the mastectomy. I did it for my children, they would say. Sometimes their words would bring tears to my eyes.

When I wasn't flashing my friends and relatives, even though I wasn't planning on becoming a swimsuit model anytime soon, it was good to start feeling like a girl again. Some of my normal "girly" activities included a pedicure, some light shopping, waxing the legs, and a haircut and color.

I don't know what it is about my hair stylist's mirror, but I generally hate how I look in it. I'm not referring to her work; it's my general appearance, my weight issues and so on. I suppose the lighting contributes to the way I look in that mirror.

I had my hair done shortly before my TRAM, but I hadn't returned since having lost more weight after the surgeries. I sat in her chair wearing a strappy tank top; the material was finished with a straight line across my chest to expose my skin above the horizontal line. Upon seeing my new braless breasts, I began noticing another change in my body as result of this surgery.

When you have your original breasts, there's a natural slope as your chest meets up with the fullness of your breasts. Looking into that mirror, I began noticing a slight cavity that was formed where that gradual slope used to be.

I couldn't wear a bra yet; certainly not the under-wire bras to which I was accustomed. It hurt too much. In any case, I didn't need a bra yet; everything was still tight. Before the surgery, when I would arrive home, the first thing I did was take off my bra. It always felt so good to let the girls loose to relax the remainder of the evening.

But after the TRAM, it felt as if my breasts were in a constant state of bra-ness. They were tight and held up higher than they have been in years, sans bra. It's a strange feeling and one you have to get used to.

Months later, when I looked at the photos from Jesse's Bar Mitzvah, these chest cavities were more pronounced than ever. I wanted to wear this beautiful gown that better showed my thinner body, but I hadn't realized how odd my chest looked in it. Naturally, perhaps this self-consciousness comes along with having a mastectomy.

Even as the muscles began stretching and I was able to stand more erect, I found I would tend to hunch over a bit and wear baggy tops that wouldn't reveal my breasts that appeared to me as odd and unnaturally shaped.

In any case, life had to move forward. I learned to adapt to these peculiar changes as they melded into who I became. When I wasn't anxious to leave the protection of my house and preferred to remain out of view of critical eyes, it was my family who made sure I got back into the world to experience some fun. As usual, it was mom who made sure there were plenty of activities for her two grandchildren while I recuperated.

One of the many gifts my parents gave to my children that summer was sending Jesse to a week of Nike Swim Camp at Stanford University. Mom was convinced our young man would go to the Olympics some day and wanted to be sure he had the tools to succeed.

I was excited he would be training under Stanford's swim coach Skip Kenney. I took a swim class from him when I was attending graduate school at Stanford and his coaching skills were marvelous. He could watch you swim a couple of laps across the pool and then pick out tiny elements of your stroke to change, resulting in your time dropping significantly. I knew he would work wonders with Jesse who was already growing into a skilled swimmer.

While I missed him terribly while he was away, I also wanted Jesse to have his first experience of living on a university campus.

By the end of the week, the first thing he said was, "I want to go to school here." That was worth the price of the camp if it instilled that drive to carry him into college. He also came home with more prizes. There were hundreds of kids attending the swim camp that week and my son managed to be one of only a few recipients of the coach's award; Jesse returned home with a medal reflecting his dedication. Then, a week later, Jesse's times dropped at the huge annual RESL meet in El Cerrito.

That summer, mom also arranged for the family to go see *Man of La Mancha* at the outdoor theatre on Mount Tamalpais. I hadn't been to that outdoor amphitheater in a few decades. Both my sisters had their graduation ceremonies there after finishing at Redwood High School.

Man of La Mancha is one of my favorite plays; I always cry at the end. But that day, I wouldn't be the only weepy fool in the audience. When she saw the musical would be playing, mom was also thinking about Sophie, our budding actress; she would enjoy the play because she loves musicals and singing. That summer she was performing on stage as a singing street urchin in *Oliver!* at Santa Rosa's Sixth Street Playhouse.

Also, thanks to mom, there were more outings planned. *Spamalot* was playing in San Francisco; mom and dad took me to see the fantastic play. Indeed, it was so spectacular, Mark took Sophie to see it another weekend. (Mark genuinely needed a hearty laugh. I talked him into splurging for the expensive tickets. After all, laughing is good for your health and soul.)

During the play when they showed the giant Star of David up on stage, little Sophie got all excited. She jumped up, pointed at the gargantuan prop and called out with glee, "Look! It's a Jewish star!" Her enthusiastic reaction attracted a few extra laughs in the audience that afternoon. Mark managed to get center seats that were six rows from the stage. Even the guy at the ticket booth was amazed they got those marvelous seats at such a late date.

As another fun outing, periodically Mark would take me to the hardware superstores in our town. These visits ensured I would walk around as I thought about new projects for the house (to be completed at a much later date, of course, if ever). This may sound odd, but I love walking through hardware stores and seeing all the fun gadgets I can use to create something. Moreover, during the summer, these locations offered a pleasant stroll through the garden centers to see all the beautiful flowers in bloom that would have been planted in my garden if I'd had the strength.

At the end of these days, when I was able to fall asleep in bed, I had begun to sleep on my side again. Rolling into that side position remained a difficult task, but once I maneuvered my body with the assistance of a king-sized body pillow to hold onto, I managed to find some comfort after my stomach and muscles relaxed into position.

Regardless of our noisy Lucy "the bitchy, old, fat cat" screaming her meow in the hallway, generally pain woke me up every half hour or so; then, I would have to switch sides. Still, being able to sleep in a reclined position again was a treasure.

Most nights, I couldn't fall asleep before 1 to 2 a.m. When you take pain meds for a long time, it tends to steal your slumber. That's what my sister told me; she's particularly familiar with the impacts generated by too many months of consuming a constant flow of pain medications.

CHAPTER 24:
REGRET OR DELIGHT?

You know how people talk about the age of their infants in terms of weeks or months for the first year or two? Obviously, part of the reason is that the baby has yet to reach a significant age worthy of a description in years; but I imagine people continued with the monthly description beyond a year because they weren't sure if their infant would survive the first year or two.

I sort of considered my TRAM recovery in that chronological fashion. I counted the weeks and eventually, those would build into months. It was right around 15 weeks after the surgery when people began asking me whether I felt regret or delight about my choice. If I could turn back time, would I do it again?

I don't know why, but the question took me by surprise. I'm glad I did it. It had been more than three months since I had my big surgery and I must say, as difficult as the recovery was the first month, I would do it the same way again.

Of course, what else was I going to say at that point?

Still, this surgery was a good solution for me and my situation. I felt fortunate I had more options than my sister was given.

As I drew closer to four months, there were many times when I noticed the movements and activities I couldn't perform. Lifting requires strong stomach muscles and I was told it takes about a year to return to normal. Regardless, it didn't feel like it would ever return to normal.

Or walking up hill, for instance, was another difficult task. Just like we had done a year before, we took a week in August to return to Hendy Woods for some camping. We hiked some of the same paths up hills as we had done in 2008.

But after the TRAM, by the time I reached the hill's half-way mark, I was holding onto my stomach. It's not that holding my belly did anything to offset the growing ache; it served more as a counterfeit panacea to stop the muscles from increasingly tightening with each step up the hills. But I didn't care. I was glad to be out of the house and camping out in the woods.

And if I'm going to be honest about everything, I have to admit another change in my body; one related to sexual pleasure.

I didn't jump back into anything sexual for many months after this surgery. Frankly, I was afraid to. And yet, when I was brave enough to try out a little sexy fun for the first time, as cautiously as I approached post-surgery sex, I found that the tightening of my stomach muscles added some extra pleasure during an orgasm. Yet, I remained guarded so as not to pull any muscles out of whack as my body naturally reacted and tensed.

Okay, that's all I'm going to say about that. If ever there were a time to accept the doctors' standard line, "everyone is different," it is in regard to sex after a TRAM.

As horrible as this TRAM recovery may appear, this was a good "lazy" way out of having to find prosthetics, dealing with ongoing implant maintenance, and more issues. Being a mom of two young kids, I didn't have time for repeat surgeries. It was done and I could move on. And what the hell; I got a much-needed tummy tuck out of the deal.

But there are times when I look in the mirror at myself and wonder how I could have mutilated my body this way. Still, it wasn't long before I had trouble remembering what my old, saggy "mom boobs" looked like prior to receiving Dr. Foster's perkier pair.

And since my surgery, now I have become living proof of the crude slang term for breasts: headlights. Absent nipples or areolae, the circular scars remaining on my breasts in truth *do* look like headlights on a car. I suppose that's my way of laughing at myself. If I didn't find something funny in my situation, surely I'd go crazy and slit my wrists or something. I figure, it is what it is.

And fuck it! I made my choice. Now I get to *live* with it. Yes, I get to live, and more importantly, I don't have to be suspended in a constant state of worrying about getting cancer. Even my kids have gotten used to the whole new tit thing and think nothing of seeing mommy walk around nude with my scars and new breasts hanging out.

But I know there are women who don't like what they see in the mirror. I have a friend who had the TRAM surgery and said she was glad she had this type of breast reconstruction because the tummy tuck improved the image of her clothed body. Still, when she is naked, she said she can't look at herself in the mirror. Seeing all the surgery scars is too upsetting for her.

In other words, as much as I hate repeating the surgeons' favorite line, it does hold true that everyone will react individually to their outcome. Of course, it doesn't hurt to have an excellent plastic surgeon. Therefore, do your homework if you are having breast reconstruction.

Consequently, should others in the breast reconstruction boat have a TRAM? It can be a good solution if you don't mind the recovery time, the scars and the long-term effects of moving muscles around in your body (you won't be doing as many, or any, sit ups in the near future...oh, darn!).

I wish the best of luck and peace of mind to anyone facing this difficult decision in choosing your favored reconstruction option (if you *have* options, that is). Just remember, when you are so confused about your options and can't make up your mind, you can always try what I did.

"Everyone vote," I told my family at one of the TRAM pre-op appointments. Yes, after a full day of medical appointments, including Dr. Foster drawing on my chest, we ended up in the exam room trying to settle on a reconstruction option. I was so befuddled by what path to take; I simply couldn't make one more decision and offered up my body's future on the back of a vote.

Each option was offered as my family, Dr. Esserman and her intern raised their hands in favor of the TRAM Flap surgery. Well, mom didn't like the long surgery, but she understood my reasons for considering a TRAM.

Honestly, the vote didn't matter; I think I already knew what I would do. I just needed some positive reinforcement to prove I wasn't crazy for choosing such a barbaric surgery.

But once the choice was final after months of oscillating determinations, no more life-altering decisions had to be made. With the recovery improving over time, I became too busy living my life to wonder about my choice.

August and September brought several weekends with Sophie being on stage in her *Oliver!* performance. My father was reasonably healthy again, and our family celebrated mom and dad's 52nd wedding anniversary. There were guitar and piano lessons in Santa Rosa, and daily swim team for the kids.

Late summer meant the county fair was in town. One of my paintings won "Best of Medium." It was an acrylic I had painted from some photos we took during a past cruise to Mexico.

And there were so many preparations for Jesse's upcoming Bar Mitzvah. My friends and family know how much I love making creative invitations, and this festive day would be introduced by a spectacular, boxed invitation.

In keeping with the ocean theme, I chose beautiful paper stock and accessories. Over the years, our family had collected shells from various beaches we had visited. Each invitation was adorned with one of those shells attached to two shades of blue vellums torn to look like waves against the sand-colored, textured card stock. The invitations were stunning and a reflection of how proud we were of our lovely boy.

My extraordinarily generous parents played their vital role in the success of his reception and more (thanks, mom and dad; couldn't have done it without you). All the while, my creative mom remained by my side as we made all my grand ideas come to life. We even had live goldfish swimming around in tall vases glowing with submerged blue and aqua lights under a layer of clear stones.

The closer we came to the date of Jesse's Bar Mitzvah, my glass-half-empty brain worried that my dad wouldn't be around (okay, yes, I mean he would die) to see his only grandson stand up at the bimah in front of the Torah at our synagogue.

Generally, a Bar Mitzvah is held near a boy's thirteenth birthday. Well, Jesse's birthday falls in the middle of December right when the cost of any party items (music, food, venue, etc.) increases or even doubles in some cases. We couldn't afford those doubled fees. Moreover, we had family from back East who would fly in for the big weekend; we didn't think it would be fair for them to pay the higher airline prices typical of the holiday season. Therefore, the rabbi agreed that we could move the date into January to help keep these costs manageable.

It was stressful enough arranging a grand event, but with every passing day, I would call my parents repeatedly to make sure my dad's health was still okay. There had been growing issues with his kidneys, and I kept telling him how he had to stay alive for Jesse's

Bar Mitzvah.

Thinking back, this prodigious milestone served as dad's carrot of encouragement on many occasions when our family wanted to give him an incentive to eat healthier or take better care of himself. And as the day drew near, too many visions flashed through my "what if" brain.

I know it's terrible to admit, but when your diabetic, ailing father is about to turn 80 around the time of a big event, you start wondering if he will end up in the hospital or die before the day arrives. Is that terribly selfish to reveal? I just didn't want anything to go too horribly wrong. I wanted Jesse to remember his Bar Mitzvah as a wonderful, joyous occasion, and not the time when he had to bury his loving grandpa.

Okay. I got that out. Well, he did survive. Adding to the festive occasion, we even got everyone in the reception hall to sing "happy birthday" to dad as an early acknowledgement of his February birthday.

I know my dad won't be alive for my children's weddings. Therefore, I'm happy he was able to participate in this celebration. This isn't being callous; it's reality. Anyway, he got to see his very prepared grandson read his long Hebrew portion.

Jesse looked so calm up there reading in front of the congregation. Many other family and friends had their parts as well, but not everyone did as well as I'm sure the rabbi hoped they would have.

My sister said she could manage to read a longer Hebrew portion out of the Torah. But she had been preoccupied by her studies and painting since returning to her apartment in Los Angeles. I'm happy her life was improving and she was back in school studying in a new field. Unfortunately, she ended up reading from her notes instead of out of the Torah.

The Hebrew in the Torah doesn't show accents, which makes it more difficult to read. When Michelle became impatient by her dyslexic, stuttered reading and switched from the Torah to the piece of paper, I watched the rabbi's face transform into frustration. I felt bad because I had promised him, my Torah readers would do just that: read from the Torah and not out of a book or off a piece of paper. Later, Michelle said she hadn't had enough time to prepare for the longer portion.

Other than Michelle's reading, only one more incident caused the rabbi to drop his head and shake it in disappointment. When my cousin went up to the bimah, his phone rang in the middle of his prayer. This is a big no-no in a conservative synagogue where I wasn't even allowed to videotape the service because no electronics are allowed.

To his defense, my cousin is one of the many doctors in my family, and he was on call. Thus, you can't fairly blame him. Maybe he couldn't leave it on vibrate. Anyway, this is *my* family we're talking about and shit like this happens all the time. Our family isn't perfect, and we all have our moments.

Other than those scene breakers, the service carried forth. In front of the rabbi, our congregation, our family and friends crowding the synagogue's sanctuary, I stood before my son. Mark stood behind me, and my parents stood behind Jesse while I told my son how fortunate I felt to be with him to witness and share this day.

"When you become a Bar Mitzvah, you become responsible for carrying out the commandments; becoming a Bar Mitzvah connects you to your Jewish history, culture, faith. Those are the elements that bind you to your past and have led you to this milestone," I spoke to my son.

"I want you to look out on all these faces. It is these people—family, friends—who will embrace you as you approach your future."

I told him how when I was 12 and had been preparing for my own Bat Mitzvah, everything changed in one passing moment. After his auntie Renee had died, my view of God, faith, religion changed and I told the rabbi, I no longer wanted a Bat Mitzvah. I became more of a cultural Jew rather than being a spiritual Jew.

It wasn't until Jesse was born and then old enough to attend school when his bubby and papa stressed the importance of religious school and the immersion into his culture, history and language. Jesse thrived at the religious school.

"Your father and I are so very proud of your dedication and effort. We want *you* to be proud of your achievements," I continued.

Truly, after my own shaky religious beginnings, I said I never expected my children would grow up with much "spiritual" awareness. If it weren't for his bubby and papa, likely Mark and I would not have put him or his sister into religious school.

"But then, this year, another significant change took control of our lives when I had major surgery. If it weren't enough that the surgery would last more than 10 hours, the worst of the recovery time would last at least 3 months," my little helper knew this story well. "As I'm sure you figured out, mommy was terrified of the surgery, the pain, the extensive scars, the continued potential for cancer, and more."

As chance would have it, something small yet wondrous happened after a Shabbat service one night in the very room where we stood, I told him.

I had been talking to a couple who became my instant friends because of common bonds with this surgery. It was during a conversation when the rabbi approached us with concern, I told Jesse. "Before I knew it, the Rabbi made sure I knew I wasn't alone; our family didn't have to face this challenge on our own: meals, rides, whatever assistance we required to make it through that difficult time over several months, the synagogue—the community—was here to help. *And they did!*" I emphasized.

I told him there were many people who offered help in various ways. Then, I asked the question, what's the point of this story?

"Through that surgical experience, I realized, we have a community. Again, look out at all these faces and you will find out, these are the people who comprise your community; Jewish and more. These are the people who bind you to your past and connect you to your future. What's more, as the descendent of Scottish kings on daddy's side, you are doubly blessed with a rich, diverse culture.

"As you stand before the Torah, you become connected to your Jewish culture, history, beliefs, laws, faith. And how lucky your community is to have you—my mench of a son—as a member of the next generation of Jews.

"Upon learning about the challenges we've faced this year, the rabbi told me, he understood the significance of the quote I put on your Bar Mitzvah invitations."

I repeated the quote by Albert Einstein who said, "Learn from yesterday, live for today, hope for tomorrow."

I told Jesse, instead of using a more common Hebrew prayer on the invitation, I chose that quote because it summed up our family and what I wished for him and his future.

"Enjoy this day; this experience. As papa says, you'll remember this always. As for your future, while life can change in an instant, it is my hope you will go forth with passion and verve."

I ended by telling Jesse, "I'm proud of you, my beautiful,

intelligent, kind, caring, considerate, sweet, helpful, thoughtful, mischievous, pensive, inquisitive, creative, loving son."

There might have been a few tears on the faces of our guests that glorious day.

I must say, in all the times my family has attended Bar or Bat Mitzvah celebrations, I've never heard a rabbi express such kind words. I'm sure many people must say that about their child's celebrated day; but truly, I was moved by what he said.

He told how in all his years as a rabbi, this was the first time he trained a student from beginning to end. Generally, there are Hebrew tutors who will help a student train for their Torah portion. In Jesse's favor, because of changes at the religious school with the dropping enrollment reflecting the poor economy, it became the rabbi's task to train our son.

That Saturday morning at Jesse's Bar Mitzvah, he told my son and everyone attending how delightful Jesse had been as a student. Just as our son was learning so much from the rabbi, our rabbi enjoyed the fulfilling experience.

He spoke about how he got to know our family better. He told about how his role as rabbi changed and grew to be more accepting of the different approaches people may have to practicing Judaism. Then, referring to a conversation I had with him on one Jesse's practice days, he was glad to see our family recognized the importance of attending services.

One afternoon, I had told him how through our weekly attendance at Saturday morning services, I may not necessarily feel a connection to God, but I recognized the value in attending the service. It was a respite from the week's stress and the repetition of the service's weekly prayers became a time to let go of the daily grind.

He relayed the story about a discovery I had made. I had told the rabbi I may not go to services every week, but I would make an effort to attend periodically. I discovered the importance of stopping and finding those moments in life that can become a relief. I was surprised he spoke of that conversation, but he wanted Jesse to know that his synagogue was a place where he could find that same sense of peace and community.

After lunch and the crowd dispersed, we had a few hours remaining to finish setting up the reception hall for that evening's party. Michelle had designed an impressive amount of beautiful fish made from sparkly ribbon or cut out of foam board she brightly painted and glittered. The tropical fish and sharks were hung throughout the hall. Thank heavens for my creative family!

As we were running around putting up the final decorations, my sister and Sophie approached me. My little girl looked up at me with worried, puppy eyes.

"What's wrong?" I asked with concern.

"I don't want you to get mad, but there's something Sophie needs to tell you," Michelle said. Sophie paused.

"What? What happened?" I asked.

"Well…," Sophie used a small voice and delayed.

"Come with us. We need to show you something," Michelle said.

The two lead the way out to the foyer. We stopped just outside the hall's double doors.

"What?" I asked. Sophie sheepishly pointed to something behind me. It was the large photograph of Jesse wearing his new navy blue suit. He was adorned by the tallis (a prayer shawl) and kippah (a skull cap) we gave him special for his Bar Mitzvah. My beautiful young man stood with his confidence and warm smile locked in a precious memory. Offering a naturally glorious backlight, the late winter afternoon's glow was diffused by the synagogues stained-glass windows and cast a luminous accent of cobalt blue tinting his cheek.

"What? Is there something…." Just then I noticed the problem.

On the wide mat surrounding the photo, Sophie had used one of the blue pens strung to the framed photograph's stand to write a message. In large lettering in a prominent position right above the photo, Sophie had written, "I wish you a bad day." I knew she increasingly had been growing jealous of all the attention showered on her brother, but I was angry at her for carrying out this spiteful act.

In the months leading up to the Bar Mitzvah weekend, mom and I continued to reinforce how Sophie would receive as much attention if she chose to have a Bat Mitzvah. Mom distracted her by taking her shopping for pretty gowns for the different events occurring throughout the weekend. Simultaneously, looking far into the future, I kept reminding her how she would get even more attention from mommy when I planned her wedding that will be spectacular and gorgeous.

"You'll do that for me?" she asked again and again as Jesse's weekend neared.

"Yes, of course," I reassured her on many occasions. Through the process of planning Jesse's Bar Mitzvah, I had already begun forming ideas using her interests as the foundation for themes at her Bat Mitzvah. She got excited every time we spoke about those ideas, but soon she would forget and begin crying as presents were sent to the house or I had to focus on the final details of Jesse's event.

And now this: a nasty message written boldly above her brother's head. Mark asked later, aren't you glad we protected the photo with the frame's glass? You bet. There wasn't enough time to have the custom photo mat replaced. Nor was there a spare photograph if she had chosen to add devil horns or other graffiti.

What could I do with this nasty message and my jealous girl?

"Sophie, why did you do this? That was such a mean thing to do. This is something we're going to save forever with everyone's happy wishes, and you had to write this nasty comment? Would you want your brother to do this to something of yours?" I wasn't loud, just saddened by her mean-spirited action.

"No," she started crying. I just looked at her with disappointment and shook my head. She began crying more with sudden remorse expressed in her eyes.

My mom walked over to see what was happening. "Oh, Sophie, what did you do?" She was surprised at her granddaughter's action.

"What am I going to do with this? I can't leave it that way, and I don't have time to do anything about it," I complained.

"Okay. Don't worry. We can fix this," mom said. "Here." With that, she grabbed the same blue pen and transformed the "bad" into "beautiful" and added a big flower, using the stem from the letter "d" as the base of the giant bloom. In the end, it still looked a bit odd, but significantly improved and less conspicuous.

Sophie's little revenge move wasn't the only hiccup, it turned out.

As with most significant events, there's always going to be a few snags. Just before the reception began, the balloon lady had to race back to the hall to replace one of her giant octopus displays right as the guests were arriving. And I was disappointed the caterer turned out to be a bit of a disaster.

She forgot drinks at the lunch directly after the morning service and a few key serving items at dinner. Her staff sucked, and they weren't attentive. Her buffet displayed no style, and at the last minute, she subcontracted the lunch to another caterer who was horrible. (My advice: be extra diligent about checking up on your caterer's skill, even after you taste their delicious food at a bridal fair.)

I know that sounds like a lot, but I don't think most people caught on to many of the mistakes and everything else was wonderful. The DJ was fabulous, and the euphoric smile on my son's face was as bright as a star when he was surrounded by his friends and family on the dance floor.

By the end of the night, after everyone had left and we remained to collect odds and ends to bring home, we were all exhausted from the fabulous party.

After nearly all the weekend's events had ended, only the Sunday morning brunch remained. Along with my parents, friends and family from out of town sat around the table and reminisced about all the great moments. Mom kept bringing up the disaster caterer until my cousin from Florida said to drop the subject. Soon, all the family would leave. We could return to normal.

Unfortunately, "normal" meant I really needed to get a job.

CHAPTER 25:
LIFE MOVES FORWARD

Following the Bar Mitzvah, I was still riding a wave of accolades from guests who enjoyed the party, the decorations, the attention to detail (that is, the details in my control).

Moreover, most of the family and our friends had not seen me since before my surgery. It was nice to hear their compliments on how I looked. They weren't just your average "oh, you look great" compliments offered as polite conversation; no, nothing like that. Instead, their faces revealed a true, happy surprise to see how I had recovered and was transformed into my thinner, new-boobed self.

It was after seeing the photos from the Bar Mitzvah when I noticed how much my body had changed. I mentioned earlier, back in June when I had my hair cut for the first time following the TRAM, I had noticed the odd indentations in the area located directly above my breasts.

Eight months following the reconstructive surgery, any swelling was gone from my torso. Looking at myself wearing a gown in the pictures, I noticed those concavities had become more pronounced revealing the absence of former cushioning from natural breast tissue.

Prior to my son's big event, I had ignored these depressions when I would wear strappy tank tops. Sleeveless tops had become the common uniform to offer relief during hot flashes.

My Southern husband tells me, women from the South refer to a hot flash as their own personal summer. Perhaps that's why First Lady Michelle Obama tended to wear sleeveless dresses and tops. The news repeatedly focused on her common choice to go sleeveless. It's my theory she was perimenopausal and wore those sleeveless tops to cool down quickly after a hot flash washed over her body.

After the Bar Mitzvah and during my ongoing battle with menopause, I continued to wear sleeveless tops even though I became a little self-conscious of this shapely change, these indentations, situated above my breasts. A year and a half after they cut out my ovaries, I became more accustomed to the hot flashes that seemed to assault my mind and body less frequently. They continued to strike the hardest at night. I find it amazing women get any sleep while suffering through menopause.

By the end of that January, reality kicked into high gear. My dad's body finally reached a tipping point and he had to begin dialysis. Once again, my mother's life was turned upside down as she entered a new hell of caretaking.

After all the years of battling diabetes, mom went with dad to his appointment and was told this dialysis was considered his disease's last stage. Dad's doctor asked if he wanted to continue the process that would require him to go to a dialysis center three days each week and sit in a chair for four to five hours each time.

"What happens if I don't have the dialysis," dad asked the doctor as though his physician's question was backed by alternative treatments.

"You die," the doctor told him. He added how he wouldn't want to be on dialysis if it were his choice. *What a shitty thing to say to a patient.* Needless to say, my parents weren't exactly thrilled with this doctor who appeared to be encouraging my dad to roll over and die. Evidently, he didn't know my father very well.

There were those who considered a kidney transplant, but that wasn't an option for dad. Aside from the likely outcome of dad dying on the table because of all his health issues, my 80-year-old father said he would refuse any such offer. He said he thought it was wrong to offer a kidney (or any transplanted part) to someone old when it could provide the gift of life to a young person.

Making the 25-minute drive to the dialysis center each week did nothing to relieve my mother's stress and she became increasingly upset about her caretaker role. She was tired and determined to make a change. Dad agreed to try a home-dialysis system that would require mom attend extensive training. There was also a surgery for dad to install a necessary port; and if everything worked properly, dad would have many more hours of dialysis time at home.

They liked the idea of the home dialysis because it would allow them to travel. Unfortunately, repeat blockages and other complications forced them back into the dialysis center.

Meanwhile, after nearly 11 months since I had my TRAM I was doing pretty well. Gosh, that actually sounded uncharacteristically optimistic. But really, my health was okay. Otherwise, everything else is relative.

Why relative? I wasn't as bad off as the people who experienced a huge earthquake in Haiti that left too many people homeless or dead, but I also knew my family needed to make some financial changes.

Between the surgeries, the long recovery and planning the Bar Mitzvah, I had taken off too much time from working. Our finances were suffering resulting in our lifestyle becoming frugal. We live in California which is a very expensive place to reside. It's easy to fall behind in bills while living expenses continue to skyrocket.

Just in time, I was hired to write online (and later, a special Sunday paper section) for the Press Democrat. I would work for this New York Times daily for two years. Not long after the paper was sold to some Florida investment group, I left the paper.

It was a dream to be working for the paper. If only the income was as rich as the experience. They paid almost nothing to the writers of our section.

Anyone who goes into journalism is told very early on, you don't become a writer to make the big bucks. I wouldn't have minded so much if it hadn't been for Mark's work.

After KRON filed for bankruptcy and cut his hours during that year of restructuring the television station, I needed to make more money to help pull us out of our debt. The station's troubles resulted in a significantly smaller paycheck which couldn't cover all the medical debt we had accumulated.

Actually, his paycheck is considered large in most any other place except pricey California and maybe New York City. And even with my new income, we began falling behind every month. I really didn't want to fall into that sad category of people who were losing their homes. And I certainly didn't want to move in with my parents! They were sweet to offer, but I hope it never comes to that.

Enough frustrating financial crap. Now, for more recovery details by the 11-month mark.

Attack of the phantom nipples, stabbing pains and make-me-crazy itching:

In the fifth through seventh months after my TRAM reconstruction, the "phantom nipples" issue escalated creating an amplified itchy sensation that couldn't be assuaged.

Mostly, my new breasts were numb. And yet, it still felt like nipples remained, especially when they should be reacting to various conditions: cold, arousal, and so on. Even when I ran my hand across the scarred mound, I still had the sensation the nipple was reacting.

Moreover, there I was nearly 11 months after my breasts had been gutted during the surgery, and I still experienced some of the "let down" nursing sensation just as I did when I had natural breasts. It wasn't as strong as before, but even nine years after I stopped nursing my children, the thought or sound of a baby crying could still trigger that mental sensation of my breasts filling with milk.

As for the itchy feeling, even though my stomach and breasts were numb, there were a few months when everything was itchy, uncomfortable and irritated. Unfortunately, scratching the numb surface didn't relieve anything. It was enough to make anyone crazy with frustration while trying to satisfy that deep itch that wouldn't cease.

That deep irritation mostly subsided by 11 months, but periodically it would return with a vengeance along with sudden, sharp, stinging feelings I referred to earlier as the jellyfish stinging. Either sensation would send me to my room where I could beat on a pillow to relieve some of the frustration. I figured, striking a pillow was better than ripping off a layer of skin with my fingernails.

Caring for fading scars and stretching stomach muscles:

While the scars remained red or a faded pink, they lost most of the knobby texture they exhibited several months before. Throughout those many months, I continued massaging the Neutrogena Hand Cream into all my scars every day after my shower. By 11 months, my scars mostly flattened out.

It took several months to be able to sit up straight absent significant pain. But nearly a year following surgery, I still experienced tightness in the muscles running from my stomach up to my new breasts. If I tried stretching my arms up too high, it felt like a spring that has been stretched a tad too far; pain would sharply strike the muscles and I was forced to hunch over quickly to avoid experiencing lingering discomfort for anything longer than a few moments.

Lifting:

Periodically, I'd try lifting a heavier item, and the repositioned muscles would snap. I mean, it felt as if someone reached inside my stomach, grabbed hold of the muscles and wrenched them, causing me to bend over in pain.

Here's a tip for TRAM patients: if you do lift something, face forward at the object. Don't try to twist your body around to your side to pick something up or you'll end up suffering; I found that out the hard way.

Standing still, and moving too much or not enough:

Standing still for longer than a few minutes continued to be difficult and tiring. Moving around was okay, but standing in one spot for too long was exhausting. The longer I stood in place, the more I'd feel discomfort increase in my abdomen and travel up through my torso. Conversely, if I moved too much through exercise or hiking up hills and other previously regular activity, my stomach muscles began hurting and tugging, causing me to hunch forward.

Sitting for too long creates its own issues when you try to stand up. I like sitting with my feet up when I watch some TV or read in the evening. I had to be careful not to sit on my side, otherwise, when I got up, I'd feel the stomach muscle pulling painfully when I rose to my feet.

If I had been sitting at my computer in the kitchen, when I got up from my chair, my posture and slow, upright recovery resembled those museum cave men displays; the exhibit that shows a succession of photographs demonstrating the evolution of man as he slowly erects into an upright position.

The point is, rising to my feet from any sitting or lying position would require an adjustment period. Otherwise, you guessed it: pain!

Learning to roll with it:

My stomach TRAM scar still made sleeping an odd experience. I had to be careful about how I flipped over from side to side. It was no longer something that occurred naturally in my sleep. It took more attention and caused me to wake up numerous times throughout the night.

If I moved without care, I felt my scars tugging. Sometimes it felt as though the scars would rip open; this was particularly true where the long scar ended on my hips. I learned to roll over as one unit instead of rolling in a snakelike movement with my legs first and the torso following. This snakelike movement required too much stretching of the stomach muscles and would result in sharp cramps.

As my skin loosened, those scar ends—one more than the other—had turned into something strange. If you've ever done any sewing, the end resembled a corner seam that won't quite lay flat. It's nothing noticeable when wearing clothes, but it has turned into a small chunk of skin protruding from my side.

Getting sick:

Coughing and sneezing remained painful. The swine flu swept through our home and coughing became a distressing procedure. With every cough, it felt as though someone was punching me in the chest and stomach. Getting sick with a cough indubitably became something to avoid; my OCD reached paranoiac levels as I tried to avoid becoming ill.

I was extra diligent about washing my hands, avoiding getting too close to people who displayed signs of illness. I suppose the latter preventative action held little value considering I've been told by doctors, by the time someone is symptomatic, generally it's too late. The period just before a person becomes symptomatic is said to be the most contagious phase.

Regardless, after the TRAM, if someone I was talking to appeared sick, I didn't feel obligated to remain a polite distance from them; I would back up and avoid contact. Getting sick equated with pain. And it wouldn't end when the cough subsided. When I wasn't suffering through coughing sessions, the sore stomach muscles would ache. I would brace my arms across my chest, but that action did little to help prevent the pain.

The times I did get sick, I found a silver lining. One benefit of having a numb stomach is it allows you to bring down a fever without experiencing the usual suffering. Let me explain.

If your mom is anything like mine, when we experienced high temperatures when we were kids, mom would lower our fevers by patting our hot skin with a wash cloth dampened with water and rubbing alcohol. After wetting our skin, she would blow air on the dampened region to cool the skin and reduce our fevers that would reach 102 F or higher; that act created pain on the hot skin.

Understandably, we hated this procedure, but she would continue until our fever broke. Every time, she was successful at her task.

Now with my numb stomach, I can decrease fevers by placing my hands (chilled from cold water) on my numb belly. As long as I keep my hands within the numb region, I don't feel the aching resulting from the temperature contrast against my hot skin. And then, my fever breaks.

Breast shape and tightness:

Several months earlier, I noted the tightness of the breast skin and how it felt similar to wearing a tight bra. Mostly, that feeling remained, but it slightly relaxed nearly a year after the surgery. I don't know if I can attribute that relief to time, becoming accustomed to the new breasts, the swelling having melted away, or a combination of all three.

Chest hair?

When the stomach skin is exposed within the circular scars on your breasts, you're left with this patch of skin that is a bit different from your natural breast skin. After all, the new breast skin comes from a different part of your body. While the natural breast skin is soft and smooth, the belly skin tends to have a bit more texture; this stomach skin also has more hair.

When I would run my hand over my skin, at first, I thought the different texture had to do with the positioning of the skin. I would compare this to texture in a piece of material; because of the direction of the material's weave, if you don't pay attention to that weave line when you are sewing, the result can look rather odd to the eye.

But after a morning shower, I realized it was more than the texture of the skin that was different. Indeed, most of the texture resulted from the hair on the stomach skin used in the breasts. Hair covers most of the body's surface, and the stomach region produces fine hairs that are slightly coarser than the nearly invisible breast hair. It's nothing like coarser leg hair after a few shaves, but that minor difference is enough to produce a sensory transition as you run your hand over the skin of your new breasts.

Weight gain and scars:

Another thing I've noticed since my stomach was stitched up from side to side is that when I gain even a pound or two, I can tell right away. The skin around the long scar becomes stretched tight like I've just eaten an enormous Thanksgiving meal. And if I let my weight climb a little more, my stomach skin begins bulging out on either side, above or below the scar. It's not pretty and motivates me to get on my treadmill.

Fanny pack bulge:

Another strange thing I noticed occurred when I leaned over at the waist. While the TRAM took most of my belly fat, when I leaned over, it seemed as though the muscles would bunch up inside my chest and abdomen. It felt as though I was bending forward over the pouch of a fanny pack wrapped around my waist. I would feel the muscles repositioning and trying to find a comfortable spot. This was a peculiar and uncomfortable feeling.

Emotionally:

Once in a while, I still question my choice to have this procedure, but I imagine time will remove those doubts as life takes over. The kids have grown accustomed to my strange body. My daughter calls the design of the scars a smiley face: the circle scars on my breasts look like the eyes, the belly button scar is the nose, and the waist TRAM scar reveals the smile. I wonder if my son will grow up thinking a woman's natural body is strange after seeing my thrashed form?

Finally, some TRAM Flap humor:

My family knows I'm terrible at retelling jokes, but here's a little TRAM Flap humor I heard from a friend:

When I winced and placed my arm across my breasts, my kids asked me what was wrong. "It's okay," I told them. "I just have a stomach ache." Ha!

Chapter 26:
A Year and a Day

It was very late when I was working on the computer and my husband walked into the kitchen. He looked at the calendar and asked, "Isn't there an anniversary coming up?"

Crap! Did I forget our anniversary? My parent's anniversary? After all, I'm the keeper of the dates in my family. I'm the one who calls my sister and mother to remind them of upcoming birthdays and notable dates; I tell my sister to call our dad on Father's Day, and I remind my mom to call her sister when it's her birthday.

"Don't you remember?" asked Mark.

"Remember what?" Should I sneak into the other room and fill out a greeting card to my hubby for something?

"Don't you remember where you were a year ago?"

Pause. "Oh, right. My surgery." How time flies.

So, there it was, a year and a day after my big surgery and I was doing pretty well. Most of the time, I felt okay. Of course, as soon as I wrote that, a stabbing pain shot through my newish right breast.

Newish? Yes, it's sort of like what to call a home's roof in real estate; one year isn't quite new enough to say it's new, thus they call it newish.

Furthermore, what do I call these mounds that were taken from my belly and moved up to my chest? They're not really breasts; not even "breast implants." Rather, they're more like heavy mounds of flesh, but saying that to people leaves them disgusted and attracts odd expressions. For this reason, I must call them "breasts."

So, what was it like a year and a day after my TRAM? At the age of 44, I felt dreadfully old. But I'm not old enough to feel old.

Unfortunately, when your body suffers every time you get up out of a chair, you begin to feel old. It's those darn stomach muscles keeping your tit skin alive that must stretch out each time you move.

This especially occurred at night when I surgically removed myself from the computer and tried to catch a quick show on television to get my mind off my writing before attempting to go to sleep. I would leave my kitchen office and collapse in the living room lounge chair that had come in so handy after my surgery. I watched TV for a while before attempting to detach my ass from the recliner. That's when the severe pain would strike.

I noticed I began staying up later and later into the wee hours of the morning to avoid the nightly routine that offered no incentive to rise from my chair.

Each night, I would have to prepare myself before standing up. I knew the pain would strike as soon as I would begin to stand. I'd clench my teeth and wince as the muscles responded to the motion that was supposed to be common. *Don't stop in the middle; that will make it worse.*

Once I stood up in a hunched position, I would momentarily pause before slowly stretching upward into a mostly-erect posture. I would brace my forearm against my belly as though I had grabbed hold of a pillow when I tried to get out of my hospital bed the year before. And when I took the first few steps, I looked like my 80-year-old father when he climbed out of a chair. Actually, he wouldn't wince.

I tried changing chairs, but that didn't help. The anticipated pain was one of those things I became accustomed to experiencing at the end of a long day. I wondered if that misery would eventually abate or become intensified.

On this anniversary, Lilly called for a chat. I reminded her of the milestone. Just like me, she couldn't believe a year had already gone by since that horrible surgery that seemed more like it happened only a few months prior.

I knew it was useless, but even after a year passed, I told Lilly how I would catch myself questioning my choice to have the TRAM and remove my breasts. Those moments of weakness retreated into the dark shadows of my self-doubting/self-loathing writer's mind when I thought about the future that likely would have been stolen had I not faced my body's cancer reality.

With this new year on the Joey calendar, I was hopeful to

attract meaningful changes in my life. I wanted to finish a book I'd been writing, and I wanted to improve our lives in the next post-surgical year.

CHAPTER 27:
WHAT'S ONE MORE SURGERY?

It's been nearly a year and a half since I had my big surgery and it appears there may be a complication that could require an additional operation.

Yes, it's my nature to see the worst in any situation before going toward the light and struggling to find the positive side. Positive side, hmm. I'm trying. Well, first an explanation.

Enough time has passed with everything healed up and scarred over. Still, the Frankenstein train-track lines that cover my skin periodically trigger surprise when I see them reflected back at me in the bathroom mirror. Those are the moments when I finish drying off my freshly showered body, remove my towel and stand motionless. I'm stunned as I look and think, *that's not me.*

It's more than simply aging and not recognizing the old face looking back at you in the mirror. These are moments filled with flashes of self-doubt about my decision; I had allowed doctors to slice me open and steal parts of my body just to leave scars and nearly square mounds of heavy flesh where my supple, natural breasts used to be.

Most of the time, I ignored the scars. Yet sometimes, like a night when I was watching *Boardwalk Empire* on HBO, it was difficult not to miss my former mom-boobs. There was a scene with a bare-chested woman reclining in bed. I imagine, because the show is set in the Prohibition Era during the 1920s and 1930s, they cast women with natural breasts, as opposed to the modern Hollywood boobs that don't move, jiggle, or sag.

As the woman on the screen shifted to lie on her side, her young breast gracefully moved with her rolling body; the supple breast changed shape as she turned over. I noticed the areolae and nipples on her breasts. Tears welled in my eyes at the thought of my mounds of flesh absent these naturally lovely creations. I thought about how no man could ever look upon my chest with the same desire as they would at this woman's ordinary breasts. I flashed back to my mini-nervous breakdown after seeing the photos of mangled reconstructed breasts on that horrible DVD I watched prior to my surgery.

I knew I could still get tattoos to create the look of areolae, and I could have surgery to form ever-erect nipples. Others may choose these options, but when considering my own body, those substitutes were not my idea of a reasonable alternative; this was especially true when I caught sight of the large scars remaining on my breasts. It would never feel natural, hence what was the point?

Mark tried to distract me from the woman's natural breasts. "But you don't have cancer, you won't get breast cancer, you won't go through chemo, and your hair won't fall out."

"It might be cheaper than getting a haircut," I told a frightfully bad, sick joke as my reality defense mechanism kicked in. "With our budget, why do you think I've been letting my hair grow out?"

"Shut up. You'll be here for the kids to grow up, and that's what's important," he always tosses in the "child argument" as he attempts to help me escape the dark side of my emotions, thoughts, feelings, fears, anxieties, anger, self-loathing and the general idea that I feel like a loser who hasn't accomplished anything substantial or worthwhile in my 45 years.

After all, I never did go to the Olympics as I had planned when I was a child filled with hope. Hope? Fuck hope. I live in the real world where my breasts and ovaries were sliced away because of some stupid genetic shit I have absolutely no control over.

Breathe. Back to the issue at hand. Most of the time, I don't think about the surgery and the scars. But after that short rant, I suppose it's clear. My choice to be proactive serves as a catalyst for dark thoughts; anger, fear, revulsion and confusion creep in and I'm left with private tears. Mark generally picks up on my desperate panic sessions and jumps in to remind me why I took such drastic measures to ensure my survival. *I desperately need a shrink (and insurance to cover the cost)!*

Even though my stomach fat lives in my chest, I still have to travel back into San Francisco for regular checks of my breast mounds.

Long after everything should have been healed and stretching into a more natural state, I thought I'd use this appointment to ask if I should be concerned about ongoing suffering in the stomach region below my right breast. I wanted to find out if this pain could be fixed. I returned to UCSF with mom who used the opportunity as an escape from her own life.

I hate the long drive into the city, but mostly I hate going to Mount Zion. The mere thought of that destination creates waves of queasiness after having gone through this crappy BRCA process. And walking through the doors of the Breast Care Center and into the back offices where my life was turned on its head makes me feel like I'm going to vomit.

As was customary, before leading me into a back room, my vitals were recorded in the hall just inside the door leading to the exam rooms and genetic counseling offices. I knew what to expect and sat down in the chair next to the blood pressure machine.

But when it came to taking my weight, no longer were they using the old-style doctor's scale: that nasty, lying fucker. The nurse walked me over to a new scale. Like a Murphy bed, she lowered the oversized base of the scale; a large sheet of metal spacious enough to roll a wheelchair onto (I'll need that for when my weight goes utterly out of control more than it already has).

After she zeroed the scale, I stood on the silver base. Red digital numbers showed up on the black screen. I couldn't help but burst out laughing.

You can't go by that number, the nurse told me about the red digits displaying less than 100 (no, I'm not going to tell you the amount). "We've gone to the metric system," she said while I laughed.

"That's the best news I've gotten in this place in two years," I said through more laughter.

"Do you want to know what it really is?" she asked me, attempting to place a damper on my momentary joy. *Hell, no!*

"No," I told her. I preferred to live in the land of denial for a while.

She said if I want to know the amount, simply multiply it by 2.2 to convert kilograms to pounds. Screw that! Let me enjoy that glorious low number for a while; one I hadn't seen since I was a scrawny thing back in high school when I considered my stick-figure legs as fat.

Are you in any pain today, she asked. That question always makes me laugh, or choke.

Before she left the room, the nurse had given me a pain form to fill out. It described how to consider the meaning behind the numbers one through 10, illustrating the levels of comfort to pain using faces ranging from a smile to a sad frown. I sat staring at the sheet when mom asked what was wrong.

"After what I've been through, I never know how to answer this question. These numbers don't make sense anymore because of the TRAM," I told her.

I continued filling out the pain sheet. I circled the appropriate pain description. Sharp? Yes. Gnawing? Yes. Deep? Yes. Stabbing? Yes. And the list went on. What makes the pain worse? I wrote, standing still, sitting, walking, bending over, standing up, etc. "What makes the pain go away," I read to my mom before writing and saying out loud, "Drugs!"

I removed my shirt, put on the robe that never fits me, and waited for my breast lumps to be examined by the ever-serious Suzie Eder, a nurse practitioner.

I explained about the aching and showed her the spot where it was generally focused. Not a day would go by without the pain, I told her. Mostly it hurt when I bent over to pick up something and when I tried standing up from a seated position.

When I finally get a few minutes at the end of the day to veg in front of the TV, I explained, it had reached the point that I didn't want to get up from my chair because I knew what was about to happen. When I go to stand up, I'm dreading the discomfort that is about to overwhelm my insides and cause my face to contort; reacting to the pain like someone is stabbing into my stomach with a large, serrated hunting knife.

"Well, that's not good," Suzie responded. I asked if there was anything that could be done, or if this were the way it would always remain. She ordered an ultrasound. I would need to return into the city in a few weeks for that and to see my plastic surgeon to discuss the results.

It felt as though one of the muscles they moved from my abdomen up to my chest lumps could be, basically, wound too tightly; there may be scarring causing the ongoing discomfort.

And how does one resolve this issue, I asked.

Surgery.

What joy is mine.

Upon hearing this, if surgery became necessary, I was hopeful it could be done with small laparoscopic incisions rather than creating additional jagged scars suitable for any villain to display.

I had the ultrasound during which my chest and organs were examined. And later, Dr. Foster told me, nothing unusual had been found. So now what? There was nothing they could do. I hoped time would make things better.

CHAPTER 28:
'THE BIG C' AND FEELING LIKE A FRAUD

After a hectic summer filled with activities, some travel, a little camping and keeping busy with my job, I was watching the season finale of "The Big C" on Showtime, and I felt like a fraud. Yes. A storage unit filled with gifts left by a terminally ill cancer patient to an only child, her son, made me feel like a fraud.

I know it's just a story on TV, but the show captures what many families—many women—go through when cancer strikes. That storage unit represented all the moments in a child's life the mother was going to miss because of cancer's dark grip and callous lust for murder.

But there I was. I had gone through this horrible proactive prophylactic process in an attempt to eliminate the possibility of cancers from my life, and as I watched the story of Cathy Jamison, I felt like a fraud.

I didn't have breast cancer like my dad's mother and sister who were killed by this genetically-infested disease. Nor did I survive breast cancer twice as had my living sister. We'll never know if my eldest sister would have gotten breast or ovarian cancers because she was killed long before the age when she could have had any form of our family's version of the "Big C."

Often, my mother has commented, had Renee gotten the same aggressive cancer as Michelle, likely she would have died. Mom guesses Renee would have had it years before Michelle did, and the treatments wouldn't have been as efficacious. Maybe that's why she was taken at such a young age, mom convinces herself. Maybe Renee would have suffered a long time before dying in the end. At least hitting her head and instantly dying was a quick end in comparison to suffering from cancer.

No, I didn't have cancer. Regardless, surgeons advised, it would be optimum for my health and future to eliminate my cancer factories; to cut off my tits and strip away my ovaries before slicing open my belly like some gruesome torture scene from the Dark Ages. My nightmare had not included chemotherapy, rather required maneuvering body parts under the protective skin of my torso, all resulting in a long recovery.

I saved myself, and yet, it wasn't because I had cancer like too many others; like this Cathy Jamison character incredibly acted by Laura Linney.

I can't say I've experienced the emotional range my sister has been forced to contend with throughout her cancer treatments and recoveries. I've had my insane moments, but my experience, my future, is opposite of my sister's story as she lives on her own and is only responsible to herself.

Still, I know how it feels to want to say "fuck it" to the world; that's how I felt when it seemed my only options were 1) you need to be sliced apart and put back together, or 2) you're likely going to get one or both of these aggressive cancers (if not some other random cancer). So, you may as well kiss your life, your peace of mind, your husband, your family, and most significantly, your children goodbye if you avoid reality and allow your body to turn into a cancer time bomb.

Wait! Can't I be like those lifelong chain smokers who never get cancer? I know that option wasn't in my cards.

My sister has had a few of those "fuck it" moments, but her episodes in hell appear more serious than mine.

Periodically, throughout this process, I had wanted to hand over all the thinking to someone else; there were too many crucial decisions to make and too many unknowns.

Clearly, I was still dealing with those unknowns 18 months after my big surgery; but as my mother often reminds me, I've never faced what my sister has.

My interpretation of mom's message is, no matter what I've been through, I don't have the right to complain. I wrestle with her dismissive message.

Nonetheless, I hope I'll never reach the same depths of depression as my sister. Like the moments just before she was rolling into surgery for the first of numerous times 15 years earlier; a memory that remains suspended in my mind when I face trials of life.

My parents had left the curtained area where Michelle lay on a hospital bed. Mom was crying and my parents feared the worst. I was about to join them, but my sister told me to wait and pulled me close to her face that suddenly turned red and contorted by crying. As quietly as she could manage through tears, she said she didn't want to wake up from the anesthesia. She said her life was useless. She felt no one needed her. It wasn't that she wasn't loved, rather, she didn't feel needed.

At the time, she made me promise I wouldn't tell our parents any of that conversation. I hated these promises. These conversations that started with "Don't tell mom and dad, but...," always ended badly. Prior to the several hours of waiting for her to wake up and before we'd hear grim news from the surgeon that started her battle with the big C, Michelle bestowed that burdensome message on me, her younger sister.

Before she was rendered unconscious for what she had desired to be the last time, I knew I had only moments to transform her determination to die; she required a longing to survive. A negative mindset is an unhealthy approach to entering any surgery. I had to convince my sister not to give up. I looked into her eyes and spoke quietly to avoid our parents from hearing.

"*I* need you," I told my pain-in-the-ass sister with whom I've always had a rocky relationship. Her tears flowed like streams when she heard my words, but she looked up at me with intensity. The terror and loss in her eyes warmed slightly with my reassuring and heartfelt words, but I knew she still might give up the fight.

Mom will go off the deep end if she loses another child, therefore you *cannot* give up, I sternly ordered. You are loved by your family, and you cannot give up. You *are* needed, I emphasized. Her face had begun to relax before they came to wheel her away. When she looked at me as they took her out of the room, I feared it would be the last time I saw her alive.

Once she was out of the pre-op room, I couldn't suppress my tears. I cried for my sister's agony and loss; I thought about our dead sister Renee and knew I wouldn't be able to recover from another sister dying. I couldn't bear being left alone.

I remained in that room, standing in the space where her bed had been only moments before. I tried to pull myself together. I had to calm down before facing our parents. And until the moment the surgeon told us, she made it through the surgery, all I could hear were her words; her determination to die.

We all blame her depression on the cancer devouring her insides. Her big C was depriving her body of energy and consuming her spirit during that time when she had what's commonly described as cancer brain.

A dash of brazen with a cup of guilt

All these years later, I sat in my living room crying after watching Cathy Jamison's scripted son discovering this storage unit filled with gifts meant to fill a future absent a loved one. I imagined other real cancer victims who had done something similar for their children after finding out they had a cancer that could not be defeated. I felt sad for those families and guilty for being emotionally torn by a process that could be the thing that, in the end, saves my life; saves my children from walking into a storage unit filled with gifts left by a mother whose body would have been ravaged by a predestined cancer if not for these potentially life-saving surgeries.

I didn't go through what Cathy Jamison did. I didn't experience anything like my sister's cancer. I didn't die like my father's family did. I found a way to spare myself and those closest to me the anguish that accompanies the big C.

And yet. I felt like a fraud.

Every time I must explain to someone why I took such extreme measures when I didn't have cancer, I feel this twinge of embarrassment. I just want to hide away from the confused stares. When people, strangers, say it looks as though I'm in pain, I want to disappear into another life, another body, and again I question my preventative actions.

I reinforce my choices calling on my high odds of getting cancer because of my mutated genes. I try not to think of that tiny chance that breast or ovarian cancers may have never entered my life. If I allow myself to ponder those miniscule odds, I may just go mad considering a full spectrum of "what if" scenarios. I must reign in my active imagination; otherwise, I'll disappear in my mind and away from living life.

I must not get angry because I was told to do pilates to build up my core prior to my surgery; the activity which messed up my shoulder (rotator cuff). When my shoulder popped during that damn plank position, that motion terminated my swimming. I guess losing my favorite exercise was the tradeoff for eliminating these cancers.

I tell myself, fuck that storage unit filled with presents to a child who isn't going to grow up with a mother who has terminal cancer. It's a fantastic, sentimental display of love by anyone who finds themself in a similar situation wherein death is imminent, but I'm not filling up a storage unit any time soon with presents to my children; let's hope, I now never have to because of the choices I made.

I did what I thought was best so I can live to watch my children live their lives. I did what I had to so I can be there and *hand* presents to them at birthdays, holidays, graduations, weddings, the birth of their children, Mother's Days, Father's Days, wedding anniversaries. I will witness them going to their proms, driving for the first time, heading off to college, falling in love, experiencing the world. I plan on being around to witness all of those special memories. And if necessary, I'll be there to show my love and support on the days they find themselves in a hospital making the same decisions I had to.

I did what I had to so I can hug them on all their momentous days, or simply because they walk into a room.

Does that make me a fraud for having not been challenged by breast or ovarian cancer? My body may reveal similar scars, but I'm not a member of the cancer club, and I hope never to be included. I just wish I didn't feel thoroughly guilty every time someone finds out about my surgeries, says "Oh" with sad eyes before assuming, "You had breast cancer?"

CHAPTER 29:
CATCHING STARES AT MY SCARRED BREASTS

I used to be a person who could care less about changing in front of other women in a gym's locker room. After all, I was raised in a household where it was natural to walk around naked. My children have been raised the same way.

My mom is an artist who paints nudes. I used to go with her to drawing classes when I was young. Moreover, her aunt lived in a nudist colony, so you get the picture (but don't try too hard because it generally wasn't a pretty sight; most people are much more attractive with their clothes on).

I had broken my foot over the summer during a family vacation. That injury and the resulting surgeries kept me off my feet for many months. Too much time passed since I maintained a regular workout and I was finally getting my ever-widening ass back in the pool. But because of my shoulder injury I still couldn't raise my left arm without pain.

That meant I was generally restricted to the back stroke and using my own oddly-designed arm strokes until my shoulder motion returns. My stroke is especially comical when I only use my healthier right arm to swim a lap.

And then, when my injured, left foot begins hurting, I tend to kick more with my right foot. Therefore, when I swim my absurd version of a backstroke, some might mistake me for a stroke victim when I give my left side a break. Doesn't that sound attractive?

As my body continued expanding, it would seem the most attractive thing about me became the cane I used. I was hopeful the swimming would change that. It's rather surprising how often I was complimented for my purple cane that has red and violet flowers on it. Yes, it's a real ego booster when the only thing people notice is the stick that assists your pedestrian abilities.

Sadly, I even reached the point that when a friend I hadn't seen in many months offered a hug and remarked that I looked good, it took me by surprise. In my own anti-social, awkward manner, I whispered in response (we were in synagogue for Yom Kippur), "No I don't." She smiled and walked to her seat. That damn "attractive" cane left me distrustful of any such compliments.

I felt quite ashamed. What a bitchy thing to do. I wanted to apologize to her after the service, but my dad was tired from dialysis and wanted to leave.

I suppose my suspicious response was all part of my "I feel like shit, I'm a failure, and my life is going nowhere" pity party. I thought I had hit another wave of my mid-life menopausal crisis.

Sorry, got distracted again; back to the gym.

Since the TRAM surgery, before heading to the gym, I started changing into my bathing suit in the privacy of my home. Once in the pool, I would swim a pathetic 26 laps. Down from my former 80 to 100 laps, 26 seemed to be my body's limit before my foot began to swell and throb with pain.

After a few minutes sitting in the Jacuzzi, I returned to the locker room hoping there weren't too many women around; especially the young and fit women.

Still wearing my swim suit in the shower, I only rinsed off the chlorine and waited to take off my suit at the locker wherein my towel awaited. Unlike before the TRAM, I began hiding my body under my towel as I peeled off my wet swim suit. Making this process more ridiculous, my OCD fears played with my mind every time the towel threatened to fall on the dirty floor. *Eew, shivers.*

But then, when I nearly fell over, I finally realized, the struggle with the towel was absurd. *Just take off your bloody suit without trying to hide.* It's not as though I was trying to show off my body; I faced the lockers like I normally do and began the usual battle to escape the dripping, snug lap suit with its crisscrossed back straps.

The day I decided to forego the semi-privacy offered by my towel, sitting on a nearby bench was a middle-aged woman who was spreading lotion on her legs. As I pulled down my black suit exposing my breasts, the woman's expression altered when she took a second look at my chest.

With furrowed brow, she made no effort to conceal her

shocked expression as she cocked her head and stared. She looked directly at my scarred tits, clearly noticing their absence of natural features.

Her reaction wasn't quite the shock factor from seeing the "Elephant Man," but certainly more than looking at Michael Jackson's final nose creation.

Realizing she was staring resulted in my tugging and tearing to escape my wet bathing suit, and quickly pull on my shirt and hide my scars from view. If I had been thinking quickly, I would have looked down in shock and exclaimed, "Oh shit! What happened to my tits?" Maybe next time.

Finally, I managed to step out of the one-piece suit when she noticed I saw her expression as I grabbed for my towel. She finally turned away, looking down at her own legs again trying to act as if she hadn't noticed anything. I caught her looking again. Her head was down, but her eyes momentarily glanced upward to stare at my breasts. *Geez, lady, why don't you just take a fucking picture!*

I wanted to hurry out of there. I dressed quickly. I sensed I was being watched by the other women in the locker room as I rushed.

These are the times I wish I didn't have to deal with, but I knew there would many more similar experiences in my future. I don't want someone gawking at me. I'm actually surprised she didn't ask about it. I think that would have been better.

CHAPTER 30:
MY FIRST BRA

"Everyone I know who is close to my age is dying or is dead already," my mom says periodically. Friends, relatives; they seem to die in waves. And late summer 2011, our family's matriarch died. I mentioned her earlier: the cousin I referred to as Golda.

Golda was strong and opinionated. She was smart, caring and one of the most generous people I've ever known. She was my mom's first cousin and they had grown up together, always remaining very close. My sisters and I also grew up around Golda, her husband and their four children.

We loved going to their house when we were young; especially when we lived in cold South San Francisco where the fog rolled in over the hill from the ocean every afternoon. They lived in Mills Estates and then Hillsborough where it was always warm, and we could swim in their pool. Golda kept refrigerators outside where she stocked sodas and ice cream; items mom generally kept out of our house and away from our diabetic father. There was always an endless supply of food at Golda's house.

I mentioned earlier, her husband, Noah, is our family's doctor. There are other doctors in the family, but none as skilled as Golda's husband. Noah was never like today's doctors who race in and out of the exam room while barely looking at your face.

Noah is old school; he takes an interest in you as a whole, not just the sore arm or an upset stomach. And it was his meticulous expertise and brilliant mind that created his reputation as a highly-regarded and skilled physician.

Golda and Noah were the first to be with my parents after Renee died when they drove my grandparents to our home that night.

And long after everyone returned to their lives and left our family to recover from Renee's death, it was Golda who met my mother in the city every week up at the Fairmont Hotel or in Union Square at the Iron Horse restaurant.

They would go out for a long lunch, get smashed and Golda would let mom talk about how lugubrious her existence had become after her first-born child was killed. Golda played a monumental role in my mother's survival. She would leave generous tips to grease the waiters ensuring this pair of women would be left alone while they got loud and obnoxious in the restaurant; they could say anything they wanted to each other and cry and cuss.

Golda was there for every significant life-changing event in our family. She and Noah took an active role in Michelle's cancer treatments and many aspects of our lives.

But the day arrived when Golda's 80-something body finally gave up on a Wednesday in August. She had enjoyed a very long life and touched the lives of countless people. She would have continued maintaining her active life, if not for her worn out body.

My aunt Donna had flown in to attend the funeral and she was staying with my parents. The funeral was to be held on a Friday morning, and both Mark and I drove our cars down to the Peninsula. In the afternoon, he could leave to head into work and I would drive my family to and from the funeral.

First, a service was held at my cousins' synagogue wherein the sanctuary was filled to capacity with friends and family. We sat in the back of the room and watched as family members delivered eulogies in front of the crowd.

I felt worst for Golda's youngest daughter, the third of four children and the younger of the two women. She took the lead arranging the service, burial and lunch. She spoke to the crowd through tears and anguish.

After the service, the line of cars passed down the hill and the procession made its way to the family's cemetery in Colma: a dreary, cold location. It had taken extra time and care to settle my dad into the car, thus we were at the end of the line.

When we arrived at the cemetery, we followed the cars and parked along the grass nearest Golda's grave. A crowd had already begun forming around the open hole. It was surprisingly warm in this shitty part of South San Francisco.

Sophie ran over to the crowd and found a spot looking down

into the open grave. Jesse wasn't as keen to go near the gravesite, nor were my parents. Dad didn't dare attempt to traverse the uneven lawn using his walker. He sat on the contraption's fold-down seat and watched from afar.

I, too, didn't go too close to the crowd. I looked around and quickly realized Golda was being buried only about 20 spots down from my sister. I felt ill.

Using my cane to maintain some balance on the grass that was due for a mowing, I made my way across the lawn, trying to avoid stepping on anyone's head. I apologized out loud if my step landed on someone's grave; it seemed like the polite thing to do.

When I made it over to Renee's grave, I looked at the marker lying on the ground. Indicating someone's visit, there were some stones sitting on the tombstone. Seeing her name, I began to cry as I do every time I visit her grave. I miss my sister terribly.

Jesse walked over to me.

"You've been here before, right?" I asked him.

He had. When my mom's aunt died I brought him over to the gravesite to "meet" his aunt Renee.

"Do you remember who this is?"

"That's your sister," he said.

I wasn't trying to test him. I just wanted him to remember where she was buried.

I don't visit her grave as often as my parents do. Every year, mom and dad bring her a cake and a beer. They light a candle for her birthday. Generally, mom would forget to buy some flowers, and then she'd steal a few from other gravesites to bring them to my sister. We're not a delinquent family; it's just that when Renee was alive, she had a thing about taking restaurant menus and ashtrays. And that was while she was attending excellent high schools in Hillsborough, and then in Marin County when we moved north across the Golden Gate Bridge from South San Francisco.

Jesse put his arm around me. "Are you okay?" He was concerned about his mommy whom he had watched cry so many times the past couple years.

I pulled him close and hugged him tightly. "You're such a good kid. I love you so much. Yeah, I'm okay. It's just hard to be here."

Mom walked over to us. "Do you know who that is?" she asked Jesse with the same intention of reminding him of an aunt who once lived. "She would have adored you," mom told her grandson. She had the same distant gaze as I; flooded by memories from Renee's short life and that horrible day we buried her in that dark trench.

As we walked back toward the crowd around Golda's grave, Jesse walked with me. As though I was highlighting different neighborhoods in the city of the dead, I began pointing to different areas of the cemetery where various relatives were buried. "Bubby's parents are over there, and that's where my grandmother's sister and her husband are."

"I know, mommy. You told me last time," Jesse said.

I didn't want him to forget these people. Otherwise, they would just become like those anonymous family members in photos when you can't remember their name or how they are related. I didn't want him to forget my sister; my beautiful, charismatic, popular, caring, generous, devoted, mischievous, loving sister.

When people saw I was crying, they thought I was doing so for Golda; and I was. Nevertheless, it was my sister's grave that elicited most of my sorrow. After all, Golda was in her 80s and my sister's life was taken much too soon.

I returned to the road to stay with dad who appeared tired and grey. We hated being at this place. Mom joined us, and we three chuckled as we watched Sophie enthusiastically throw several handfuls of dirt down into the grave onto Golda's casket.

"Oy, look at your daughter," said mom.

"If she falls in, I'm not jumping in after her," I said.

Before retrieving a small bottle of champagne from the car, mom waited for the funeral to end. Golda loved a glass of champagne and mom wanted to share one last toast with her cousin and dear friend. Some relatives noticed what mom was doing and said they wished they had been equally prepared. "Aw, that's perfect for her," a cousin said.

After the funeral, the family and friends returned to the synagogue where there was a catered lunch waiting. Mom fell in love with this caterer and told me how we should have had this woman cater Jesse's Bar Mitzvah.

"I got her card," mom whispered. "For the next event."

The remainder of the afternoon was spent schmoozing with relatives and friends who were visiting from all over. As usual, my family was one of the last to leave. Mom was busy catching up with relatives who had flown into town. And she spoke with Golda's children (the youngest is older than I am). She wanted to find out the plan for caring for elderly Noah who would now be living by himself.

He was still practicing medicine—likely will until the day he dies—but he was terribly unsteady on his feet and hard of hearing. Mom knew Golda would want her to make sure the kids were watching out for their father who would be alone after too many decades of companionship.

Aside from the sadness brought on by the day's somber occasion, there was something strange in the air; a sense of significant change.

For years, Golda had been the one who brought the family together for the High Holy Days or her annual July Fourth barbecue. She brought all sides of the family into her home. Now, it felt as though that was changing. No, it was disintegrating. Golda always took care of this and more responsibilities for the family. Until this funeral, none of her children took up the task of these family gatherings. I felt as if this were the last time we would all be together.

For many years, Mark and I would hold summer barbecues at our home. We don't have a pool like Golda and Noah did, but we still invited the relatives. Some years, we would join forces with mom and dad and have the party at their home; they were located a half-hour drive closer to the cousins. Still, only the youngest daughter and her family would come. She made the effort. On rare occasion, and only when the event was held at my mom's home, her older sister would make the drive north for the parties. I think it was my mom's garden tea party she attended.

It's sad when a family loses that connection. One of these days when my parents are gone, I know I'm unequivocally going to feel cut off from my family.

It was growing late, and most everyone had left. We walked out to the parking lot with a few remaining cousins and said our goodbyes. Before leaving for work, Mark brought my car over to the curb where we had maneuvered my dad into the front passenger seat. Everyone else climbed into the back of the car.

The ride home was loud, as usual, while mom, her sister and I chat on about the day. Mom expressed her worries about Noah being alone; she raved about the caterer and gossiped about the family. There were no rests in the conversation all the way back to Marin where we stopped at the Cheesecake Factory for dinner.

The restaurant is at the Village Shopping Center where there is a Nordstrom's and Macy's anchoring the ends. For several weeks, mom had been telling me about this bra she had begun wearing.

"Joey, they measure you for the perfect fit, and it isn't one of those underwire bras that hurt so much," explained mom. There had been many years when mom stopped wearing a bra, but suddenly, she found it comfortable to wear them again. She thought this bra would offer me the same comfort.

She knew I hadn't worn a bra since the TRAM because of the pain and discomfort caused by the material's tension over sensitive areas. She watched me hide my chest behind layers of clothing, or by hunching over a bit.

"Joey, let's go over to Macy's real quick after dinner and see what they have. I'll buy you a bra," mom said eagerly at the opportunity to go shopping. Donna and the kids would come along.

By the time we walked to the other end of the open-air mall, most of the shops had already closed. Inside Macy's, there were hardly any customers as they neared closing time. We passed by the shoe department, took a left and headed over to lingerie where a woman was alone at the check-out counter.

"Can you help us?" mom asked the woman. "My daughter needs to be measured for a new bra." It became mom's task to tell the woman about my bilateral mastectomy and how my breasts had changed. We weren't sure what size bra I required. The woman appeared hesitant.

"Oh, uh, I don't think I'm comfortable measuring you," she said to me. *Crap! That's great. Am I that much of a freak?* "I'm not the regular person for this department. She went upstairs for a few minutes. But I could call her down. I think she would be able to help you better."

She called the other woman and I began wandering through the racks of frilly, flowery, lacey bras. Most were underwire bras that would dig into my chest if I wore them.

"Mom, what kind of bra are we looking for?" I asked.

"Oh, it's the one with the little pink breast cancer ribbon on it."

"Well, that narrows it down," I said, looking out at the sea of brassieres. "Are you wearing it now?" She was. I went over to her and lifted the back of her shirt to look at the tag. The print had faded.

A few minutes later, a woman, younger than the last, responded to the call for assistance. She came over to us offering help. Again, my mother had to explain why it was necessary for her to size my breasts.

The woman led the way to the changing rooms and grabbed a measuring tape. Donna watched the kids as they wandered through the racks near the changing room.

"Do I need to take off my shirt, or leave it on?" Either was acceptable, she told me. "If you're uncomfortable with this, I understand," I added after seeing the other woman's troubled reaction; but this young woman surprised me.

"Not at all. I've seen every kind of breast come through this place," she said with confidence and caring. After all, back in the 1990s, it was reported by the San Francisco Chronicle that breast cancer studies revealed Marin County as the state, nation and world's "hot spot" for breast cancer, recording the highest rates of incidence among white women.

The Macy's lingerie lady wrapped the tape around my chest and noted some measurements as my mom told her about the bra she wanted. Again, mom lifted her top to show her bra. "Sure. That's a Wacoal."

"That's it," mom said. "I can never remember that name."

"Oh, I've had Wacoal's in the past," I told her. "Lilly told me about them years ago." The bra is comfortable and comes with a higher price tag than most bras.

"I love the way it fits. And the straps don't fall off your shoulders like other bras," mom added.

The young woman went to an area against the wall around the corner from the entrance to the changing room and found the Wacoal bras. Unlike the colorful bras hanging on racks standing in the middle of the department, the Wacoal colors were neutral or black. They had some floral lace on the front layer, but the brightest feature was the tiny white tag displaying the pink breast cancer ribbon.

"Try these on to start," she handed me a few bras.

As I returned to the changing room, I heard mom speaking quietly, chatting with the woman about the breast cancer gene, my prophylactic mastectomy, and the TRAM surgery.

I entered the changing stall and closed the door. I took off my shirt and stood in front of the tall mirror that hung on the wall. For the first time in more than two years, I wrapped a bra around my chest and looked down to latch the three hooks. It was the correct size; not grabbing too tightly or causing discomfort around my chest. I grabbed the material at my sides and slid the latch around to the center of my back, performing this simple act I had done thousands of times since I was a teenager. As I raised the straps over my arms until they rested on my shoulders, my new breasts settled into the cups.

But it wasn't right. These breast mounds didn't fill the cups as my former natural breasts had. I tried to mold my squarish, flatter boobs into the rounded cups, but the extra material that should have been filled by my body was left deflated and wrinkled like a used balloon.

I stood there in front of that tall mirror and looked at my topless torso and the semi-deflated bra cups. I stared at the scars on my belly. I noticed the flattened area above my breasts that used to reveal a natural slope that had beautifully transitioned into my former breasts.

My sight was fixed on this false reflection. It felt like I was truly seeing my body for the first time in two years.

I had become one of those headless women in that DVD that had sent my senses over the edge into confusion, anger, loss, depression, fear, emptiness and isolation.

"What have I done?" *Who could look at such a deformed body and ever think it was beautiful, feminine? How could I have done this to myself?* Simultaneously, I thought how breasts are just piles of skin and tissue and shouldn't mean so much. *Should they?* Tears formed. I tried to muffle my crying. Mom and the Macy's lady entered the changing area and asked if the bras were fitting.

"Um. Well. Not exactly," I said through tears. Mom heard my voice and knew right away something was wrong.

"Joey, open the door. What's wrong, honey?" she asked in a soothing voice. I kept staring at my horrible torso. "Come on, sweetie. Open the door. Let me see."

I opened the door. "Oh, sweetie," she said.

"I'm sorry. It's just. I just look so horrible, and my breasts don't fit because the cups are round and my tits are square. I don't look normal. I just…I'm sorry."

"Oh, sweetie, there's nothing to be sorry about," mom said.

"Don't be sorry. I understand," comforted the Macy's lady. "I see so many women who go through the same thing." She was kind and understanding. "It's okay. You look great compared to a lot of women I see in here."

"But I don't fit right. My boobs don't fill the cups right," I repeated. By this time, Donna walked to the stall to see what was happening. The Macy's woman said I only required a different cup size. She and mom quickly returned out to the Wacoal racks to search for a bra that would offer a better fit. Donna remained and stood there with me as I dried my tears. She said she didn't understand why I was so upset and then revealed her heartless side.

"I guess you were more attached to your breasts than I would have been. To me, it wouldn't have been such a big deal," Donna offered this dismissive comment before leaving the changing area. I closed the stall door. I was stunned and angered by my aunt's callous words. I know her remark wasn't meant to injure; it was one of those "pull a thought out of your ass and speak before you think" observations; it was like when I was a kid, and I'd hear people ask about my dead sister, "Aren't you over it yet?"

I felt foolish for reacting so intensely in this public place. I was glad it was late with no other women in the changing area.

Mom and the Macy's woman were still chatting when they quickly returned. They carried more bra sizes I could try. Thankfully, the lower-sized cup fit my breasts for the most part; there was only a small amount of floppy material which I managed to shape and smooth around my boobs.

"There, see?" said the woman. "And you know what? I have another idea." She walked out of the changing area. Shortly, she returned carrying a box. "Here. Try these. A lot of women who've had mastectomies use these. We call them chicken cutlets."

She showed me how to place the gelatinous forms (yes, nearly in the shape of a boneless chicken cutlet) into my bra. "See? See how nice that looks?" She was supportive, non-judgmental and continued to offer kindness. The store was closing, but she made no attempt to rush us through this process.

"Joey, that looks beautiful," mom looked surprised and happy. "You want them, Joey?" She didn't wait for an answer. "We'll take them," she told the woman.

I looked in the mirror and saw my shape had improved. The better cups and the lift offered by the cutlets made me feel more like a woman again. "They do look nice," I said shyly.

Thanks to the kindness offered by this stranger and the wholehearted love offered by my devoted mother who yet again found a way to steal away anguish from her child, my confidence began rebuilding.

Months later, I still have moments of doubt, but a voice growing with strength takes control and I become empowered when I tell myself, *fuck it. I'm alive, and I don't have breast cancer. I don't have ovarian cancer.*

Life has continued. I still have my family, my children. I still have hope. I can look to the future absent the terror I had when I found out I carried the BRCA genetic mutation.

In telling my story, I hope other women who face this journey know they are not alone. I hope you have the love and support of family and friends. I hope you grow confident in your choices and can settle into peace of mind.

Just as I had my children to influence my decision, my choices, I hope you have something that inspires you to fight your battle to become a cancer survivor, or a BRCA genetic mutation previvor. Find that element in life that grabs hold of your spirit and carries you forth to rise above adversity and live in strength.

APPENDIX:
TRAM FLAP PATIENT ADVICE

What you want to know before heading into surgery

A breast cancer survivor wrote to me on my blog at JoeysJournal.com and asked what advice I had to offer anyone preparing for a TRAM Flap surgery. I realized, I had been writing about my experience of having this barbaric surgery, and yet I hadn't offered information about what one should do to prepare for such an operation.

Therefore, the following is my advice to TRAM Flap patients with the caveat that this information is based on my experience; it is based on not having cancer, and choosing this surgery to avoid my high chances of breast cancer.

My experience is immensely different from someone with breast cancer who may have several surgeries before, after and/or during chemotherapy and radiation treatments.

With that in mind, I hope you will pick and choose what works best in your individual situation.

Prior to TRAM Flap surgery

Choosing your surgeon

I don't claim to be an expert on how to choose a surgeon. Moreover, I must admit, I was in a better position than many people since my sister had already been through breast cancer twice and had two of the best surgeons in the San Francisco Bay Area.

Therefore, I was familiar with their work because of my family. Regardless, I still asked questions about how many TRAMs they had performed. I wanted to see photos of my plastic surgeon's work. I wanted to know the success rate of a TRAM; and I wanted to know if there were any statistics about the failures. What were the most common reasons for these failures? If the procedure weren't a success, what would happen next? What options for reconstruction remained if the TRAM failed?

As much as I was freaking out about having this surgery, I knew I had to find out some of the details. It may seem ridiculous to say this, but do your research. Know the type of work your surgeon does. Based on the various surgeons, there can be vast differences in the end results.

I suggest following the advice of a friend who was an emergency room nurse. When you want to find the best doctors and who does the best work, go to the hospital and speak with nurses. Find nurses who work with a lot of TRAM and mastectomy patients. They can't officially recommend someone, but there are ways around that as long as you don't hold them liable in any way. Ask who they would go to if it was their body going under the knife.

If you're like me (tested BRCA positive, but I didn't have cancer), you may already know you will have surgery; furthermore, you have options. This surgery process is a significantly different experience for someone with breast cancer. Like my sister, many times breast cancer patients are rushed through the surgical process and their choices may appear limited.

I had too much time and too many options to think about, but that also gave me more of a chance to pick and choose what I wanted and who I wanted to carry out the surgeries. Do your research, or have someone who isn't panicking to help you through this process.

Exercise

Once you decide to have the TRAM Flap surgery, if you are able, try doing the exercises your surgeon suggests to strengthen your core and build up your stamina. If you are in the middle of chemotherapy or radiation, it is understandable that you may not feel well enough for any exercise.

I was better at building my stamina than doing the core exercises they offered, but I'm glad I was swimming or briskly walking for an hour most days leading up to the surgery. Do what you can under your doctor's supervision. It seems to have helped me and it might do the same for you.

If you have children

My two children were still in school when I had my surgery. Therefore, they had something to do during the day up until summer vacation began when my young daughter's favorite complaint was, "I'm bored."

Still, they had their weekly activities including music lessons a 20-minute drive away. We didn't want to lose their timeslots, therefore, I made arrangements with family and friends to drive them the first month or so until I could drive them on my own.

Obviously, if you have the funds, make arrangements for summer programs at your local recreation department, sleep-away camps, and so on. Or perhaps this would be an opportune time for younger children to visit grandma and grandpa for several nights.

Otherwise, your friends and family become priceless during this time. Once the initial support system is removed from the recovery equation, I hope if you are facing this surgery, you have some loyal friends who will help with your children. This brings me to my next area of preparation.

Friends and family are priceless

It is during the month or two (or three) following your surgery when you realize how thankful you are to have friends and family upon whom you can rely. You may need to call people to help with:

- grocery shopping
- picking up medications
- driving to and from doctor appointments
- helping you shower (the first week or so at home)
- carry things, like pillows and plates of food
- cooking meals
- general errands
- helping around the house
- and more. There's always more.

Everyone is busy with their own life. While many people will offer their help when they find out you to have this significantly impactful surgery, likely many of those offers will fall through because people have their own responsibilities. Still, if you can find a few friends who can help, their assistance can make a significant difference in your recovery. Or if you belong to a church, synagogue, book club, or whatever, don't be afraid to contact them for help: meals, driving, and more tasks. You'll be pleasantly surprised by the offers of help.

In other words, try to get these things set up prior to your surgery. The better prepared you are, the more smoothly your recovery process will be at the time when you won't have the energy to worry about these things.

Items to have ready before returning home

Obviously, you'll want to stock up on everyday items such as shower supplies (shampoo, body wash), frozen meals and essential groceries. But there are several additional items (some suggested to me by others) that come in handy once you return home from the hospital after a TRAM. Here's the list:

• **Shower seat:** Especially during the first week home, you may want some kind of shower seat when you are unable to stand for long periods. They sell these at medical supply stores and sometimes at Costco or other big box warehouses. You're not supposed to be submerged in a bath until the incisions heal (not that you'd have the strength to get into or out of a tub). Once your surgeon says you can take showers, you'll find they will be exhausting at first. You'll want to sit down on something while your hubby, family, or whoever helps you wash your hair, legs, or anything you can't reach or have difficulty washing.

• **Showerhead with extension hose:** When you're sitting on your shower seat, it's useful to have a showerhead that can extend so you don't have to spend too much exhausting time standing in the shower, or sitting and fighting with the water stream. This is especially convenient if you have someone helping you wash your hair, and so on. They aren't too difficult to install, they don't have to be expensive and they make a substantial difference in providing additional comfort during showers. Moreover, the extra control over the water stream helps keep incisions drier when necessary.

• **Recliner chair:** Another friend told me about this indispensable item. If you don't already have one, purchase or borrow a cushy reclining chair of some sort. I call mine, "the throne," because I spent a significant portion of my days sitting in that chair the first six weeks at home. I have TRAM Flap friends who said they even slept in their recliners the first couple of weeks because you can't lay flat for more than a month after the surgery. I set up my recliner with an ottoman and a lot of pillows. I had a small TV-dinner table beside my chair to hold all my daily necessities: drugs, drinks, phone, etc. A couch isn't terribly comfortable, and they tend to be difficult from which to rise.

• **Armrest pillow:** At night the first few weeks, I found this armrest pillow to be extremely helpful when piling up the pillows. Again, you won't be sleeping in a flat position because all your muscles tug and it's stressful on your belly scar. Moreover, sleeping on your side is painful. I don't know what it's like for someone who has a TRAM for only one breast, but having a bilateral mastectomy doesn't leave much room for sleeping on your side. Additionally, the pillow's built-in armrests help keep your arms elevated and the weight off the sides of your sore breasts.

• **Back scratcher:** I know this sounds silly, but you can't imagine how handy a modest back scratcher is. You know the kind; the cheapo, long bamboo stick with the curled end and the jagged edge. Trust me, when you can't reach those itches on your back, that's exactly the time your back becomes itchy. In the hospital, you'll find it quite handy when no one else is around because you will have limited arm movement. Scratch your back, your leg, the back of your knee, your toes; there's always something to scratch when your body is unable to reach it (especially when you're not allowed to bathe properly, and your body becomes grimy – sorry to be gross, but it's true).

• **Back scrubber:** Just as a back scratcher is useful, a back scrubber (like the kind with a shower puff at the end used with body wash) can be used in the shower when you don't have someone to help wash those hard-to-reach spots.

The first week in the hospital

Have an advocate

The surgeons don't always tell you as much about TRAM recovery as the nurses may, and the first week in the hospital seems never to end.

For a great many years, my parents have believed when someone goes into the hospital, they should have an advocate with them. I highly suggest having someone stay with you during the first few days and nights after surgery; during the days when you are groggy from all the pain medication and may not know what you want or need all the time. I realize everyone may not have this type of support system, but if you can arrange it, you'll find it beneficial in the beginning.

Not only is it comforting to have someone looking out for you to make sure you're not given an extra dose of some medication that will cause you to overdose (that's nearly happened to me a couple times during other hospital visits), but it's helpful to have someone there when you can't move to reach something across your little bed table in the hospital room where a nurse may not check on you more than once every few hours.

Have something to do...or not

I went to hospital all prepared with two audio books on one Mp3, and hours and hours of music filling another Mp3. I knew I would be drowsy from drugs, therefore, trying to read (and hold) a book was out of the question.

In the end, it didn't matter that I brought these things. I never used them. I was in and out of sleep most of the time. Regardless, I likely would have wanted them had I not brought them. You may as well be prepared.

Also, I wanted to write whilst I lay in bed; my computer was a must. It was also rather convenient the hospital provided internet access. Looking back, I don't know how I got through some of those first blogs, and later, I noticed numerous mistakes I made. I am thankful my mom helped me prepare the photos for downloading them to my stories. (My advocate to the rescue, again!)

I didn't bother bringing anything like a sketch pad because it hurt to keep my arm raised for any length of time. And focusing on something for more than a few minutes had been excessively difficult in the beginning. In the first few days, I could barely keep my eyes open.

Don't over pack

I don't know what I was thinking, but I packed 10 pairs of undies and an equal amount of socks along with extra sweat pants and shirts. Silly me. Other than the pair of undies I wore into the hospital, I didn't wear them the entire week under the loose hospital pants. This was because the TRAM belly scar hurt if pressure from the panty elastic pressed on it. I did wear a different shirt and socks to leave the hospital, but I wore the same comfy hospital pants to go home and continued my absence of panties for a while. Otherwise, I only wore hospital gowns that first week.

Get up and get moving

I know you won't want to, but as soon as you are able, begin getting up out of bed and start walking.

It's painful and hurts like a bitch, but it does benefit your recovery. You'll be getting out of bed differently, and you'll learn a new style of moving that helps limit your pain level. You'll swing your legs around to the side of the bed while simultaneously raising your body. It may seem impossible at first, but don't worry; you will get it. Try practicing it at home prior to your surgery so you get a feel for it.

If you don't get up much, at least make sure to ask the hospital if they have one of the air mattress beds that adjust every time you move. Likely, you won't be sleeping on your side because it hurts too damn much, consequently that air mattress bed makes a world of difference on your back and buttocks.

Leaving the hospital

You'll want to have several pillows padding and protecting you from the seat belt and the bumpy ride when you are sent home from the hospital after your TRAM.

Many hospitals use disposable pillows. If your hospital uses these, only the pillow cases must be returned. Therefore, bring some pillow sheets from home to use, and then use these disposable pillows in the car. Otherwise, be sure the person driving you home brings several pillows with them in the car if your hospital doesn't allow you to take them from your room. I found it comfortable to sit on one and use two in front of me to protect my body from the tightening seat belt.

When you return home from the hospital

The first week home

You're still going to need a lot of help when you return home. My husband took off two weeks from work to care for me and our children once I returned home. He was there to help get me up out of bed in the morning and continued assisting me throughout the day. He helped with my showers since I couldn't yet reach down past my thighs to wash or dry. Also, he would wash my back and hair.

He was there to carry my many pillows from the bed to my throne downstairs in front of my computer and the television. He was there to bring me meals, drinks, and medications. He would separate the medications into Ziploc bags clearly marked with the time of day I should take the medicines; he kept track of all my meds when I still wasn't thinking clearly.

Get used to taking numerous pills every day. Don't skip your antibiotics used to avoid infection (that's how my sister ended up with one of her expander infections because the antibiotics were upsetting her stomach and she stopped taking them).

Call your doctor if the pills make you feel ill. And as for pain meds, I took mine regularly in the beginning. I had no desire to act like a hero and endure the pain.

If you're not up for reading, you may want to use a service like Netflix when you return home. The essential pain medication tended to dull my senses from doing anything more constructive than watching movies. Plan on being bored out of your mind for a few weeks.

Walk...and again, walk some more

My husband was diligent about getting me out of my throne and walking every so often. Walking around feels rather odd the first few weeks. Walk through your house and it feels as though your muscles are pulling you downward. Just keep doing it, even when you don't want to. Eventually, it starts getting easier. I hope you have someone to motivate you as I had. If you don't have someone at home to tell you, have one of your friends call you every day to tell you to get off your ass and walk. You'll thank them later.

Getting out of the house

You're bound to go nuts in the house after a week or so. If you're lucky to have someone to drive you, after the second or third week, you're going to want to get out. Take short trips to start. For me, the longest trips in the car were the 1.5-hour drives to see my surgeon during post-op appointments.

You're going to need someone to drive you around until you're off the serious pain medication (mine was Percocet). It might take you a while to build up the courage to drive yourself, especially if you have a large car/truck that makes the steering wheel a bit heavy. Turning the wheel can create sharp cramps in your chest if you follow the hand-over-hand method. I had a friend who offered to ride shotgun the first time I went out. I hope you have someone to go with you the first time, too. Oh, and don't forget your pillows!

Handicap placard

When you do start going out, you may want to ask your doctor about getting a temporary handicap placard. The Department of Motor Vehicles has a form you can bring to your doctor to fill out. (You may be able to print it out online from your local DMV site) Your doctor may say, "Gee, we don't usually get too many requests for those," but get one anyway. Yes, you are supposed to walk, but when walking through the grocery store is exhausting, you'll be glad you have it for a few months. My doctor set it up for six months.

Wheelchair and a cane

If you have access to a wheelchair, you may want to use it the first week or so when you leave your home (with the assistance of someone pushing you, of course). Borrow one if you can. My parents had a lightweight travel wheelchair that was perfect for the first few weeks home.

Otherwise, see if you can find a cane to use during the first month. They're also much cheaper than a wheelchair to purchase. As time goes on, you may not need the cane to walk as much as for when you have to stand still; waiting for an elevator, waiting for someone to bring the car around to pick you up, waiting while standing for anything. A cane provides a little more assistance when you feel as though you can't stand any longer and your muscles keep pulling you downward. Eventually, you'll need it less and less when you go out.

What to avoid

Too hot, too cold

Don't use hot or cold compresses on your new breasts or

anywhere on your skin that is numb. First, extreme hot or cold may cause skin burn when your numb skin prevents you from noticing the dangerous temperature change. More importantly, serious burns or frozen tissue can destroy the breast tissue.

Lifting anything heavy

My doctors and nurses all said the same thing. "Don't lift anything heavier than the Sunday paper." I took this advice seriously because I didn't want to create any bulging hernias. Anyway, you don't want to feel the pain it causes when you lift anything weighty. Otherwise, you can experience pain in your breasts, across your chest, in your stomach or in your back.

Don't wait too long to call a doctor

You've just had serious surgery. If you show any signs of problems related to your surgery areas, or other signs like fevers or foul odors from your wounds, call your doctor immediately. If there's excessive oozing or redness, call your doctor. Ask your doctor what to look for with regard to problems and your TRAM Flap not healing correctly. Don't be afraid to call your surgeon.

I have a friend who had a TRAM, and she thought everything was going well. Things changed remarkably quickly after she returned home. The skin began to die in one of her reconstructed breasts. That day, her surgeon removed the TRAM Flap breast and replaced it with an implant. Again, call the doctor quickly if you suspect a problem.

Don't forget to take a photo

Modern technology can be a tremendous tool. When I had problems with my new belly button, for instance, we would take a photo with our phone (or you can use a digital camera) of the area that seemed to be getting infected and e-mail it to someone at the doctor's office. Then, they could better decide if we needed to come into the city. That's better than making a long drive just to wait for a surgeon to tell you nothing is wrong.

House cleaning

Don't worry about your home or the laundry getting done. No one cares what your house looks like when you are recovering. (No one, that is, except my mother who said one day, "I hope the rabbi didn't see your house looking like this.")

Let others help you through this difficult recovery. If you don't have friends or family who can help, the American Cancer Society may be able to help with these and other tasks like grocery shopping and driving to doctor appointments.

Wait for showers

Wait for approval from your doctor to take a shower. The first week in the hospital, you'll be given sponge baths; not as satisfying as a shower, but better than nothing.

More questions to ask your surgeon

• If you require chemotherapy or radiation, there may be a waiting period before you can have TRAM Flap reconstruction. Collect these scheduling details as early as you can so you can make your arrangements with family and friends to help.

• I chose not to have nipples created, but you may want to. Find out how long you will have to wait. The same goes for areolae tattoos and when you can have those made. Ask to look at photos of how it looks on other women to determine if you want the same.

• Find out what size breasts you can have created from your stomach tissue. Be clear about the size breast you want in the end.

• Find out how properly to care for your new breasts with massage, physical therapy, and so on. What signs should you watch for to make sure the tissue isn't dying? Find out what happens to your chest if the tissue dies. If that had been the case in my situation, I was told I would have to have an implant.

• Find out where the incisions will be made and where the scars will be located.

• Find out your options if you're not sure you want to do a TRAM Flap (e.g. DIEP Flap which has a higher chance of tissue not surviving because blood flow is interrupted when the tissue is entirely detached from your body. Still, it doesn't impact your muscles the way the TRAM Flap does.). Recovery time is different for the various surgeries, therefore, do your research to choose what's best for you.

In your journey to eliminate cancer from your life, I wish you best of luck and good health.
Truly,
Joelle

About the author:

Joelle Burnette has been a writer for a New York Times daily newspaper in Northern California after having written for other newspapers following receiving her master's in journalism/communications from Stanford University. Her writing experience also extends to her work in television news in San Francisco, congressional offices on Capitol Hill and in California, and media relations on presidential and other regional political campaigns.

When she isn't writing, Burnette enjoys camping, traveling, photography, painting, swimming and spending time with her family.

Connect online:

Facebook: www.facebook.com/joelleburnette.books
Smashwords:
www.smashwords.com/profile/view/joelleburnette
Blog: www.joeysjournal.com
Follow Joelle on Twitter @joelleburnette

16615708R00167

Made in the USA
Lexington, KY
03 August 2012